Super Powders

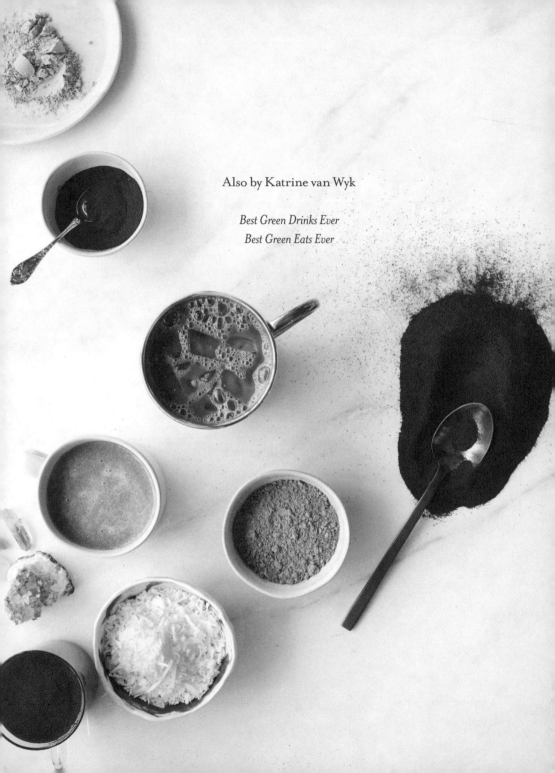

Also by Katrine van Wyk

Best Green Drinks Ever
Best Green Eats Ever

Super Powders

Adaptogenic Herbs and Mushrooms for Energy,
Beauty, Mood, and Well-Being

• • •

With 50 Recipes

Katrine van Wyk
Foreword by Frank Lipman, MD

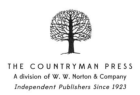

THE COUNTRYMAN PRESS
A division of W. W. Norton & Company
Independent Publishers Since 1923

IMPORTANT NOTE

This volume is intended as a general information resource. It is not a substitute for professional advice. "Super powders" (supplements that contain adaptogens) are not evaluated by the FDA and can have or cause significant physical effects. Ask your doctor before starting to take any supplement, even if you have used it in the past, and get a medical diagnosis from your medical doctor or other professional healthcare provider before you use adaptogens to alleviate any medical or psychological symptoms or discomfort. Be sure to read the author's introductory safety note for additional important safety guidelines. **Many adaptogens are not considered safe in pregnancy. Adaptogens are not recommended for anyone taking immunosuppressant medication.**

For information about permission to reproduce selections from this book, write to Permissions, The Countryman Press, 500 Fifth Avenue, New York, NY 10110

For information about special discounts for bulk purchases, please contact W. W. Norton Special Sales at specialsales@wwnorton.com or 800-233-4830

Manufacturing by Versa Press
Production manager: Devon Zahn

The Countryman Press
www.countrymanpress.com

A division of W. W. Norton & Company, Inc.
500 Fifth Avenue, New York, NY 10110
www.wwnorton.com

978-1-68268-313-2

10 9 8 7 6 5 4 3 2 1

AUTHOR'S NOTE

I wrote this book because I truly believe that learning to use "super powders"—supplements that contain adaptogens, also known as superplants and tonics—has improved the quality of my life and that they can improve yours, too. But not surprisingly, there are disagreements among doctors and others about the benefits and risks of ingesting these "super powder" supplements. Not everyone thinks it will have any effect, some caution about overdoing it, and some say that certain substances can actually be harmful. Also, I don't know how old you are, what your regular diet is, or whether you have any genetic or medical conditions or allergies. So:

- Consult your doctor before you start to ingest any supplement, especially if you are pregnant or nursing or if you suffer from any allergy or other medical condition, and especially if you are taking any prescription medication.

- Check the ingredients of any supplement you are considering using. Make sure it doesn't contain anything to which you are allergic. Also check for any known side effects. Some supplements can cause very serious reactions, including, in rare cases, paralysis and death. Others can interfere with both prescription and over-the-counter medications.

- Definitely consult your doctor if you have begun to ingest any supplement regularly, whether or not in supplement form, and you don't feel well. While there may be absolutely no connection, it's always better to be safe than sorry.

- Check with your doctor before you start to include any new fruit, vegetable, or any other ingredient from my recipes as a regular part of your diet. Some foods carry risks for some people. For example, goji berries, which I use in one of my recipes, can negatively interact with warfarin and diabetes drugs.

- For all the reasons stated above, never give any supplement to a child without first checking with your pediatrician.

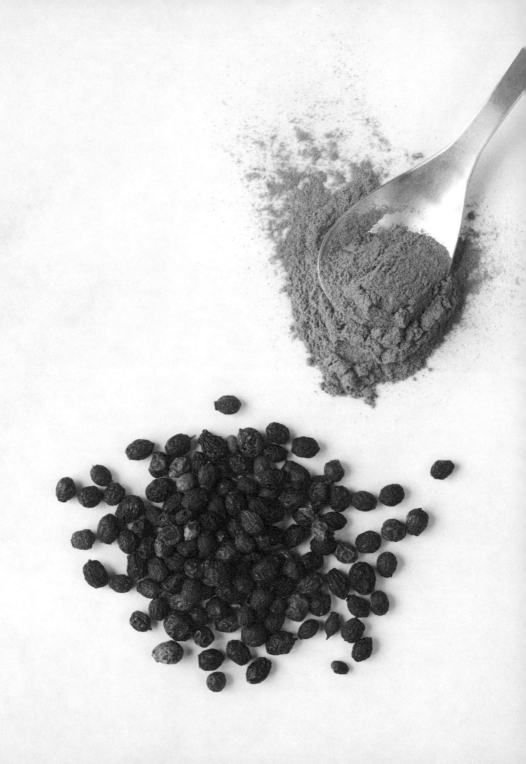

CONTENTS

FOREWORD BY FRANK LIPMAN, MD

At my practice, Eleven Eleven Wellness Center in Manhattan, I see a lot of patients who suffer from symptoms linked to or made more severe by stress and exhaustion from their demanding lives. They're often caught in a vicious, chronic cycle of too little sleep and then consuming too much sugar and caffeine to get through the day and relying on alcohol or medications to wind down and sleep at night. Thankfully, there are healthier ways to get through the day.

I believe in food as medicine, and with the help of nature's incredibly powerful super foods, the human body can do a lot to heal itself. I'm a huge fan of a unique group of plants known as adaptogens, which can be used to improve the health of the adrenal system—the system in charge of managing your body's hormonal response to stress. Practitioners of Ayurvedic and Chinese medicine have known about the power of these plants for centuries. I've trained with doctors of Chinese medicine and have used adaptogens in my own practice for decades. By supporting adrenal function, adaptogens can counteract the adverse effects of stress. They enable our cells to access more energy, help cells eliminate toxic by-products of the metabolic process, and help the body utilize oxygen more efficiently. The result is a clearer mind and more resilient body—and a better complexion. I like to think about adaptogens as working similarly to a thermostat: when the thermostat senses that the room temperature is too high it brings it down; when the temperature is too low it brings it up. In the same way, adaptogens can calm you down and boost your energy at the same time! It's quite amazing.

Katrine has worked in my practice for years, observing how amazing these plants are at helping people restore balance in their bodies. In Super Powders, she introduces readers to 25 of these roots, mushrooms, and herbs and explains how to incorporate them into their daily routine. One of the reasons that patients love her is that she is great at distilling all of the food and wellness advice out there and making it easy and clear to follow. That is exactly what she's done in this book: she's taken what is often considered stuffy "herbalist" information and pared it down to what you actually want to know about these amazing plants.

If you were worried that you'd have to swallow a capsule of powder to get the benefits of adaptogens, think again. This book is full of Katrine's signature fun, easy, appetizing recipes. Although I do believe in targeted supplementation, the complex combination of nutrients found in food makes adaptogens more absorbable in the body. These recipes are designed with just the right healthy fats—like nuts, seeds, and coconut oil—for optimal absorption.

I'm also thrilled to see Katrine include some of my other favorite super foods like turmeric, medicinal mushrooms, collagen, matcha, activated charcoal, and spirulina. Turmeric's anti-inflammatory benefits are well studied; when a patient complains about pain or is recovering from injury or surgery, I recommend supplementing with turmeric to help their body combat inflammation. I make sure to eat it regularly myself, too. For patients needing to cut back on coffee and caffeine, I suggest green tea or matcha as an alternative. And collagen is one of the latest additions to my must-have daily super powders for gut and skin health.

Good health requires one to be proactive and, in Super Powders, Katrine helps readers do just that. I hope you will enjoy studying these powerful plants and discover their benefits for yourself through these delicious recipes.

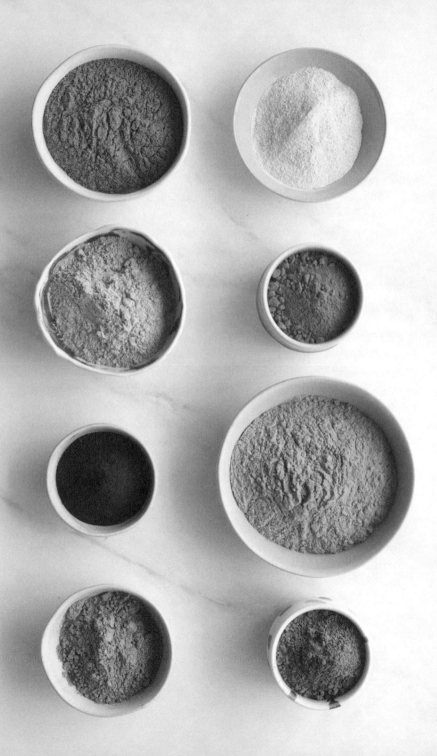

INTRODUCTION

When writing a book, I tend to write the introduction at the end. I started this project knowing that adaptogens and superfoods were amazing and could be beneficial to so many and I am very excited to finally be able to share this information with you. People need to know about the many amazing plants out there that they are not yet utilizing!

Many companies are making these plants more accessible and, frankly, more fun to explore, with beautiful packaging that highlights their benefits. They are also creating tasty blends that combine several powders for new and exciting results. I have used these adaptogens and super powders myself for years and recommend them to my nutrition and wellness clients. I have seen how wonderful they can be: these plants have the amazing ability to expand our capacity to handle any kind of stress.

Now, after completing my research for this book, I feel that way more than ever! The process of writing *Super Powders* confirmed to me how powerful, yet gentle and balancing, these plants can be. It blows my mind learning just how intelligent they are. Mushrooms may not look like much when you see them growing on a dead tree stump, yet they can have great healing benefits. Gnarled roots that may seem like ugly weeds to the naked eye have amazing anti-inflammatory, calming, or even mood-elevating effects. All of these barks, leaves, roots, stems, fungi, flowers, and berries are harvested in nature and simply powered by the moon, the sun, and Mother Earth.

Although these plants may not be a total panacea, they certainly may help prevent, relieve, and even contribute to the healing of many stress and lifestyle-related problems. People today are struggling with illnesses, anxiety, mood disorders, neurological diseases, autoimmunity issues, and cancers. Yet humans have known for thousands of years about the healing and balancing effects these plants have on body, mind, and spirit. They've been

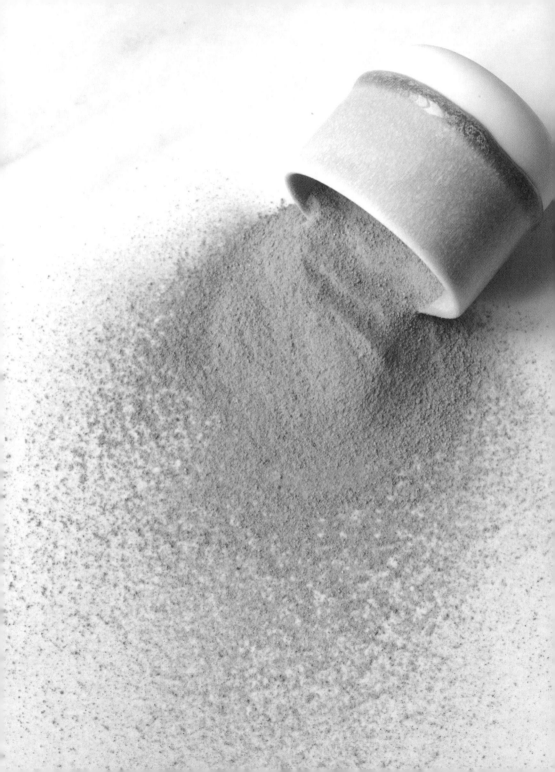

incorporated into rituals, used by royals and monks, and helped shamans and medicine men in their healing work. Now, research is confirming what they knew all along.

Please use the information and the recipes in this book as you will. Incorporate these super powders into your life however it feels right to you. Experiment. Create. Improvise. Learn and observe. Use your intuition and have fun!

With love,

Katrine

13

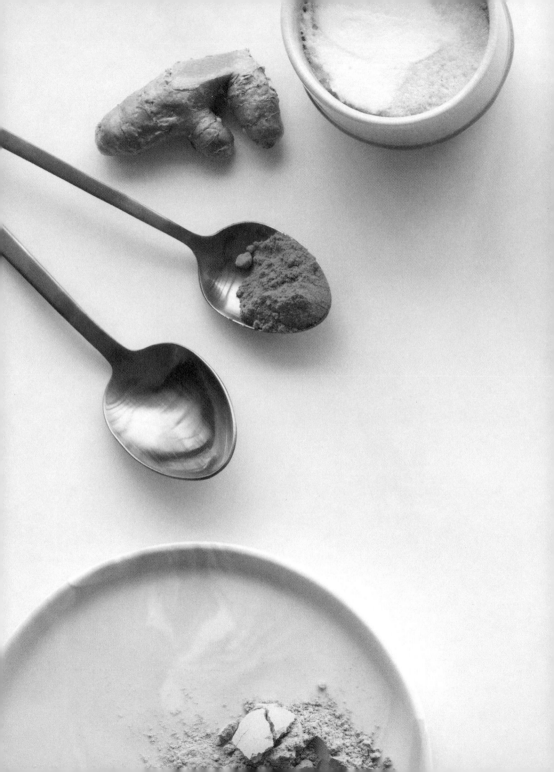

PART ONE.
INTRODUCING
ADAPTOGENS

WHY WE NEED ADAPTOGENS

We lead such busy and full lives. Our schedules are jam-packed, our vacations are too short and far between, and we're demanding a lot from our body and mind every day. What if there was something you could do to improve your performance, increase your resilience, help you sleep more soundly, and upgrade your energy levels? What if adding a few small rituals into your routine could transform your day and make you feel just a little more amazing?

A group of ancient plants called adaptogens have been utilized for thousands of years by practitioners and healers all over the world. They were used to help people who had demanding physical work or who were recovering from illness. Back then, the things that were perceived as stressors to humans were a little different than what we're dealing with in the modern world, but our body's reactions remains the same just like the amazing benefits of these plants.

Thousands of years ago, the source of our stress may have been a lurking tiger or a bitterly cold winter season. Today, it may be a screaming boss or the pollution in the city where we live. However, our nervous system is the same and our hormonal response to stress, no matter what the cause, remains the same. Adrenaline gets pumped out from our adrenal glands and causes our heart to beat faster, our mind to become acutely aware, our breathing to become more rapid so more oxygen can get to our muscles, and our blood to pump to our limbs (and away from our digestive and reproductive organs). Then, cortisol is produced and released. Often called the stress hormone, cortisol triggers the flood of extra blood sugar to give our body the fuel to run away. All these physical responses to stress prepare our body for fight or flight! This is crucial for our survival when we're in real danger and is meant to be a short-term, on-and-off response to tackle a threat. Once we're out of harm's way, our body turns off the stress response. But what happens when we're constantly stressed, running from one thing to the next? The stress response hardly ever turns off! We are stuck in survival mode: cortisol is constantly produced and released, and our blood pressure and blood sugar remain high all the time. After a while, our body can become insulin resistant, which is the beginning stage of prediabetes and eventually diabetes. Cortisol also causes our body to store fat around our belly and store extra energy as cholesterol (turns out, stress is a big contributor to high cholesterol). It can even lead to cravings for sugar, carbs, salt, and fat. Meanwhile, the adrenaline keeps us hypervigilant and makes it hard to fall asleep at night. This state of chronic stress can lead to all kinds of health problems, including difficulties with sleep, digestive issues, anxiety, brain fog, and fatigue. What a mess!

I first discovered adaptogens when I was overcoming what is often referred to as adrenal fatigue many years ago. I was depleted, burnt out, and tired all the time. Yet I was only in my early twenties! Sound familiar? Most people will deal with these kinds of symptoms at some point in their lives, but increasingly many are facing these challenges while still very young. It seems as if it is now just part of modern life. The amount of pressure we put on ourselves to be successful, as well as the external pressure we feel from society, can be overwhelming. With the demands of school, parenting, work deadlines, workouts, and even socializing, many of us feel stretched too thin and stressed out. Add the disruption and distraction of being constantly available through cell phones and social media, and it's the perfect cocktail for a system shutdown. I mean, I'd love to meet the person who isn't dealing with some level of stress in his or her life, but the reality is that most of us are juggling a lot of things at once and our body can't help but respond.

I don't accept that it has to be this way. Prevention is always the best approach! We can focus on strengthening our immune system and our resilience, on improving our ability to be the calm eye of the storm, on supporting our body to work optimally! And on tuning in to our needs, imbalances, and signals, which can allow us to get ahead of more severe problems down the line. Instead of a mind-set of always pushing harder, doing more and doing it faster, we can do things better, more mindfully and intentionally, with more clarity and calm.

Adaptogens have been instrumental to my recovery from what was both an emotionally and physically draining time (hello, fashion world!) and I'm thrilled to be able to spread the word about these superplants. I worked alongside Frank Lipman, a functional medicine doctor in New York, I saw how adaptogens seemed to be helping his patients on a daily basis. New York is a city of type A's who are always on the go, juggling lots of projects, deadlines, and responsibilities. A lot of his patients spent most of their time traveling, changing time zones weekly, while still needing to look and perform at their best. Dr. Lipman prescribed adaptogenic blends to support and strengthen these patients. Some needed a more calming blend, whereas others needed an energy boost. What is just so cool about these adaptogens is that there's something for everyone.

If you're dealing with a health challenge, I encourage you to seek out a physician or another appropriately licensed healthcare practitioner for a medical diagnosis. Once you have that, you can determine the root causes of your challenges and, working with that physician or other licensed professionals, customize a treatment plan that's right for your needs. We are all different and I firmly believe there is no one approach or answer, one set of herbs or supplements, or one type of exercise that is right for everyone.

WHAT ARE ADAPTOGENS?

Adaptogens are a group of intelligent plants that work with the body. Instead of giving the body "fake" energy surges, the way coffee or sugar does, adaptogens improve the health of your adrenal system—the system that is in charge of managing your body's hormonal response to stress. Adaptogenic plants can range from roots, leaves, and berries to mushrooms, and they can be prepared and consumed in myriad combinations. Quickly summed up: adaptogens help your body better *adapt* to stress!

Research suggests that adaptogens relieve stress by modulating the release of stress hormones from the adrenal glands. So if you're feeling overwhelmed and anxious, adaptogens can help you calm down and get grounded. If you're feeling run down and worn out, adaptogens can help get you back on your feet and ready to tackle the day again. When it feels as if life is coming at you at 200 miles an hour—adaptogens can be the trick up your sleeve that helps save the day by aiding your body in regulating cortisol levels and keeping you level-headed and calm under pressure. Adaptogens can even help you rest and sleep better so that you can perform better. Sleep is the first thing to tackle if you're dealing with fatigue, burnout, low energy, cravings, and weight gain. (Any new mother knows the feeling of brain fog and the sugar and carb cravings that come with sleep deprivation—which means adaptogens are amazing tools for new parents during this big life change. I'm not sure I would have made it through the first few months after my daughter was born, while also keeping up with my three-year-old, without my daily dose of ashwagandha).

What's truly wonderful is that these plants, aside from a few exceptions, are not stimulants like sugar, alcohol, and caffeine;

rather, they help stabilize and support your body to function well. They don't draw from your body's nutrient reserves and they won't send you on a roller-coaster ride of energy highs and lows the way other common stress aids do.

Adaptogens can help you restore balance or prevent crashing during demanding and stressful times. These herbs work with your body so that no matter how the stressors are throwing your body out of whack, they help your system seek that state of homeostasis that it craves and strives for.

Adaptogens also boost immunity, increase focus and stamina, and may reduce the feeling of fatigue. They can help increase your energy levels and even boost your mood and sex drive. Adaptogens are ideal for whoever wants to boost their overall well-being, optimize their body's function, and feel great.

TRADITIONAL WISDOM

Adaptogens have been used for thousands of years to help raise our body's resistance to stressors. Whether from our environment, toxin exposure, emotional trauma, mental fatigue, illnesses, or anxiety, adaptogens have been used as a tool to help us cope. These powerful plants have been utilized for centuries in Ayurveda and traditional Chinese and Tibetan as well as Native American medicine. Many of the same plants appear in both Chinese medicine and Ayurveda, often under different names. Adaptogens also may be referred to as tonic herbs in some books and articles, and the terms are often used interchangeably. In traditional Chinese medicine, the belief is that a person is healthy when the body is in balance and energy (called qi) can flow freely. From this point of view, disease is a state in which there is imbalance. A large number of the ancient Chinese remedies used to correct imbalances and support health are the same plants that we now refer to as adaptogens.

Ayurveda, often seen as yoga's sister, is the traditional healing tradition from India. It's a 3,000-year-old oral tradition that is still practiced and celebrated today. Ayurveda also emphasizes that health is a state of balance between mind, body, and consciousness. Many of the herbs mentioned in this book have been used in Ayurveda to help support and restore balance (including turmeric, which is *not* an adaptogen).

Traditionally, the plants were foraged in the wild and they often grew (and many still grow) in rugged, challenging terrain, just like the terrain in our lives that they're intended to help! These amazing adaptive plants often favor steep, rocky, harsh, cold climates. Many plants with adaptogenic benefits are found in mountainous regions, such as the Himalayas and Andes. Today, most adaptogens on the market are cultivated and their environments more controlled.

MODERN SCIENCE

What healers and doctors of alternative medicine have witnessed, experienced, and thought for a long, long time is becoming more and more mainstream. These approaches are now accepted as good treatments for stress-related health challenges. It is truly exciting to see this ancient wisdom get validated by modern science.

The actual term *adaptogen* is really quite new. During World War II, Russian scientists were experimenting with different substances to help their pilots and submarine crews increase their stamina. They looked to traditional cultures to see which plants were commonly used to survive harsh and challenging circumstances. For example, they learned that the Nanai hunters (the native people of far eastern Russia) used a tonic made from Schisandra berries and seeds to help reduce hunger, thirst, and exhaustion as well as improve their night vision. Later studies revealed that Schisandra indeed contains several compounds that have been shown to protect against stress and enhance cognitive function. In the 1950s and '60s, the idea that medicinal herbs and plants could increase stamina and survival in harsh environments was established and the term *adaptogen* was coined.

Today, adaptogenic herbs are even given to people undergoing chemotherapy and radiation treatments for cancer in China. Because Chinese research suggests that certain adaptogens help protect the body from the side effects of chemotherapy and radiation treatments as well as increase the patients' overall well-being throughout the treatment process, Chinese doctors are incorporating these plants into their patient care.

ADAPTOGENS WORK

The one thing all adaptogens have in common is the ability to help the body better *adapt* to stressors and challenging environments.

They work both in the immediate moment and with long-term use. Say you have a big day of work meetings and presentations ahead of you—taking some adaptogens might make you perform better, help you stay focused, deal with any stressful situations that occur, and keep your energy up! Or a cup of holy basil tea at night might help you unwind and calm down before sleep. A study of rhodiola, Schisandra, and eleuthero found that one single dose of these effectively increased mental performance and physical endurance in the test subjects! Pretty cool stuff.

In the long term, adaptogens can work with your stress-response system (a.k.a. the hypothalamic-pituitary-adrenal axis) to help your body adapt to stress and actually cause it to produce less stress hormones. The best part is, adaptogens can do all that without the unfortunate side effects of most other stimulants, such as caffeine, sugar, and alcohol (common effects of those are addiction, tolerance buildup, sleep disruption, and blood sugar issues). Adaptogens also work to regulate the immune system. Whereas some people might need their immune system to activate to help prevent them from getting sick, others may need the immune system to calm down and stop overreacting, which is the case for allergy sufferers.

Some of the many amazing benefits you may experience when introducing adaptogens to your life are:

- Improved cognitive functions: focus, memory, and clarity
- A boost to your libido, desire, and heightened pleasure
- Strengthening of your immune system—bye, flu season!
- Strength, stamina, and performance boost
- Curbed cravings
- Improved sleep quality
- Sense of harmony and balance
- Hormonal balancing
- Slowing of the visual signs of aging
- Glowing, radiant skin
- Loss of belly fat
- Increased lean muscle mass
- Boosted energy levels
- Calm reactions to stressful situations
- Support and recovery from stress, exhaustion, and exercise
- Elevated consciousness and protection of your energy and vibrations
- An overall feeling of well-being

Yes, adaptogens are amazing plants that can further your health goals and boost your well-being. They may help you snap at your kids less, focus better at work, or sleep well at night. But, as with anything in the health and wellness world, they are a piece of a bigger picture. Just taking adaptogens on top of an otherwise unhealthy and overscheduled lifestyle may improve your stress levels somewhat, but you do also need to take care of yourself in other ways! Eating nourishing, whole foods, engaging in physical exercise and time outdoors, and getting adequate sleep, as well as participating in meaningful relationships and love are crucial for a thriving mind, body, and spirit.

If you're exhausted, adaptogens will help with energy. If you're feeling anxious, they'll help you calm down. They optimize the body's adrenal functions so that you can better cope with your busy, everyday life.

REAL, WHOLE FOODS

A *lot* of potions, pills, and powders on the market promise the world. It can be confusing, overwhelming, and even off-putting at times. Aren't we supposed to get our nutrients from our *food*? Well, yes, of course!

But even though our lives today demand a lot from our mind, body, and spirit, we spend less time preparing and feeding ourselves quality food! In addition, the soil in which our food is grown is depleted of many important nutrients due to modern, industrial farming practices that grow bigger crops faster but strip the soil of its nutrients in the process. When our body is stressed and our digestion not working optimally, we also don't absorb all the nutrients we eat. There are even foods (coffee, sugar, and alcohol—I'm looking at you!) that can flush minerals and nutrients from our body! On top of that, the world—including the air we breathe and the water we swim in, shower in, and drink—is polluted. No wonder our body needs a little extra support and TLC. This is where super powders come in to play. They are real, whole foods that are simply dried and turned into convenient and longer-lasting powders, the best of them without any added fillers and preservatives. Another great benefit to adding these plants to our life is that we're increasing the variety of plants we're consuming. In the past, people would traditionally eat hundreds of different types of plants in a year, but today most of us only eat a fraction of that. Each plant contains a different and unique set of phytonutrients, so by adding more varieties to our diet, our body is getting more diverse vitamins, minerals, antioxidants, enzymes, and proteins. Adaptogen powders are derived from whole, real plants and are potent, intelligent, and amazingly effective at giving us the nutrients we desperately need!

HOW TO FIND THE RIGHT ADAPTOGENIC SUPER POWDER

The wonderful thing about adaptogens is that they adapt to your needs. And because these adaptogens will meet you where you are in this moment in time, it might require some trial and error to find your personal favorites. Many adaptogens can seem almost identical in their benefit descriptions. There is certainly a lot of overlap, but each adaptogen has its own unique spirit and personality. For example, even though two different adaptogens are helpful for sleep, one might work better for you than the other.

When you're getting started, you might want to stick to one adaptogen at a time—slowly adding it to your diet and noticing how it's working with your body. Just because an adaptogen worked well for your partner or BFF, or its online enthusiasts, does not necessarily mean it will be the best fit for you!

If you're dealing with a burnout, make sure to go with a very low dose of the gentlest adaptogens. Once you build your strength (by eating lots of nourishing food, regulating your blood sugar, and getting plenty of sleep and active rest) and get some energy back, you can always branch out and try others, carefully monitoring how they make you feel.

Although many people experience instant effects after taking certain adaptogens, it may take a while before you experience any changes. It's worthwhile sticking with one adaptogen for at least a couple of weeks before ditching it and moving to another. Of course, if you're experiencing any discomfort, such as insomnia, anxiety, diarrhea, or overstimulation, it may be a sign that you and that particular adaptogen are not the best fit for each other. Listen to your body, pay attention, and tune in! Trust your gut and intuition (and consult your medical doctor if the symptoms persist). If you align your needs and cravings with the right adaptogen, it can be a powerful tool on your wellness journey.

- Identify the challenges you have, imbalances you feel, or goals you'd like to achieve. For example, do want to calm down your nervous system? Boost stamina and strength for your workouts? Improve your erratic sleep? Lift your mood? Feel sharper and more focused at work?

- Now that you know what you're trying to improve, look through the next section for the super powders that will give you some of those desired benefits.

- Start with a small dose of one powder at a time so that you can monitor how each makes you feel. It may take weeks before you're really seeing the benefits.

A QUICK REFERENCE GUIDE TO CHOOSING AN ADAPTOGEN

STIMULATING ADAPTOGENS
Red Asian ginseng, white Asian ginseng, rhodiola

CALMING ADAPTOGENS
Ashwagandha, cordyceps, reishi, Schisandra

BEST SUITED FOR YOUTH AND/OR HEALTHY PEOPLE
Eleuthero, holy basil, rhodiola

BEST SUITED FOR EXHAUSTED AND TIRED PEOPLE
American and Asian ginsengs, cordyceps, shilajit

FIND YOUR FIT

Here are some suggestions for adaptogens to try, based on common challenges and situations:

FOR THE STUDENT

- Rhodiola: this brain-supporting adaptogen can help with memory retention, mental clarity, and improved learning.
- Cordyceps can help boost your mental power.
- Lion's mane supports brain function. It's just what may be needed to increase concentration and focus.

FOR THE NEW MOM

- Ashwagandha: in the Ayurvedic tradition ashwagandha has long been used by nursing moms to support breastfeeding. A great stress reliever that is good to take both morning and night.
- Shatavari: known to increase milk supply in nursing women. Also celebrated for being able to increase vitality and fertility.

Note: Adaptogens are *not* considered safe during pregnancy, but are generally safe while breastfeeding. Check with your pediatrician to be sure.

FOR THE TRAVELER

- Both Asian and American ginseng can help with symptoms of jet lag.
- Amla may help protect the cells from damage from radiation—a great benefit for those who do a lot of air travel.

FOR THE APHRODISIAC SEEKER

- Schisandra helps support the sexual organs. For men,

that means increased stamina and sex drive, and for women, an increase in sensitivity and circulation.

- Ashwagandha has long been believed to help increase sexual desire in both men and women. It's been used by women in India for centuries to help support their sex drive.
- Maca has been shown to improve libido and sexual function and is a great overall hormone balancer.
- Pine pollen is a potent aphrodisiac and hormonal balancer, and can help increase libido.

FOR THE SEASONAL SNEEZER

- American ginseng is known to strengthen the immune system increasing the body's ability to handle allergens.
- Licorice can help with allergies, especially sensitivities to animal dander and allergic asthma.

FOR THE "ALWAYS SICK"

- Cordyceps is known as a lung strengthener and has been traditionally used by people with asthma.
- Astragalus, when taken over a period time, can help build up the body's resistance to colds and flus.
- He Shou Wu supports immune function and is believed to help the body resist colds.

FOR THE WORRIED WARRIOR

- Reishi is celebrated for its immunity-supporting benefits as well as enhancement of longevity. It also provides stress relief and promotes calmness and centered feelings.
- Ashwagandha is one of the few adaptogens that are calming and it is amazing during trying and stressful

times. It has traditionally been used for people experiencing anxiety, nervousness, and insomnia.

FOR THE ONE WHO'S GOT THE BLUES

- Holy basil is a soothing adaptogen that can help balance the nervous system and bring a feeling of harmony.
- Asian ginseng can have an uplifting effect, is lightly stimulating and energizing, and may be just what's needed to get out of a rut.
- Pine pollen contains DHEA, a hormone that can help boost overall mood.
- Rhodiola can help reduce the stress hormone cortisol as well as increase production of the feel-good hormones serotonin and dopamine.

FOR SUPERBEAUTY

- He Shou Wu is the adaptogen for promoting youthful hair! It helps prevent hair loss and fights off gray.
- Amla is a hair strengthener that helps strengthen the roots and supports overall hair growth.
- Goji berries are packed with antioxidants, vitamin C, and beta-carotene, which help protect the skin from premature aging.

FOR THE INSOMNIAC/UP-ALL-NIGHTER

- Ashwagandha is calming and supports good sleep.
- Schisandra has been shown to help overcome insomnia.
- Eleuthero improves the overall quality of sleep and can promote sleeping through the night.

FOR THE GYM RAT

- Eleuthero increases endurance and stamina and helps with recovery by aiding in the metabolism of lactic and pyruvic acids. Lactic acid buildup is what gives you the uncomfortable heavy and sore muscles after a hard workout, so anything that can help prevent or minimize this buildup in the first place is of great benefit to anyone working out. It also supports weight loss by causing the body to use fat for energy.

FOR THE [LADDER] CLIMBER

- Schisandra enhances work performance. It promotes focus and stamina while also having a calming effect. It may help fight off anxiety so that people focus on their goals and avoid feeling down due to fears and worries.

FOR THE GENERALLY EXHAUSTED

- Rhodiola has been found to increase activity of the mitochondria (the cellular energy centers).

- Eleuthero supports stamina and endurance and increases energy.

- Astragalus can provide an immunity boost to people who are feeling run down.

WHAT TO KNOW
BEFORE YOU START

TAKING ADAPTOGENS SAFELY

What's unique about adaptogens is that, almost by definition, a plant known as an adaptogen is unlikely to be one that's known to cause side effects in most people. Of course, there are no guarantees but, in general, plants categorized as adaptogens are considered safe, nontoxic, and non-habit-forming. It's still always wise to use common sense, do your own research, and trust your body and your instincts. It is also always best to check with your physician before starting on any new supplements and herbs, especially if you are on medication or under their care for any health issues. A licensed acupuncturist that is trained in Traditional Chinese Medicine (TCM) might be a good place to start. Many functional medicine doctors—MDs who take a holistic approach—are also well versed in herbs and supplements and can work with you to find the right fit for you.

Note that even though most adaptogens are considered safe for daily use for most people, many are not considered safe in pregnancy. They are also not recommended for anyone taking immunosuppressant medication.

So, once you've consulted a doctor and/or health practitioner, it's safe to begin an adaptogen routine! Adaptogens tend to work best when taken regularly (for a period of around 6 to 8 weeks), so if you don't feel an immediate effect, give it a little time! And, rest assured, taking several adaptogens together is not only safe but also often recommended and can lead to a more balanced and supportive effect. Lots of powdered blends on the market now target different desired benefits. However, if you're brand new to adaptogens, you might want to start with one at a time to monitor how it makes you feel before adding another. You can also create your own custom blends once you know which plants work best for you.

Which adaptogen works well for you can change over time, depending on your lifestyle, stress levels, illness, and health challenges, so an adaptogen that may work well at one stage of your life might not be the best fit a few months or years later. Continue to check in with yourself about how you're feeling!

GOOD TO KNOW

- It's a good idea to rotate the adaptogens in your routine every couple of months.
- Taking a break one day a week, one week a month, and/or a month a year is also often recommended.
- Adaptogens are contraindicated with some medications, so always check with your doctor before starting to take any adaptogenetic supplements.
- Do not take adaptogens during pregnancy without a physician's okay. Adaptogens are usually *not* considered safe in pregnancy.
- Adaptogens are generally considered safe while breastfeeding and some are even beneficial for milk supply, but again, ask your doctor.
- Some adaptogens are considered safe and beneficial for kids, too! Ashwagandha may help boost their immune system during back-to-school time. But always check with your child's pediatrician before introducing any adaptogens or other herbal supplements.
- Most adaptogens can be used as single herbs, although many herbalists prefer to blend them together to create a synergistic effect.

- What works wonders for your best friend might not work as well for you.
- Adaptogens can help your body find homeostasis and balance, but may still not treat a chronic, underlying issue or medical condition.
- There is no substitute (or super powder) for proper rest, sleep, and nourishing food!

YOUR ADRENALS, THEIR STRESS RESPONSE, AND CHRONIC STRESS

We can't really talk about stress and adaptogens without first understanding the adrenal glands and how they respond to stress. The adrenals are part of our body's endocrine system (also known as the hormonal system), which includes the thyroid and reproductive organs. The adrenal glands (there are two) sit right on top of the kidneys and are responsible for regulating our stress response by secreting adrenaline and cortisol. They usually do this in a rhythmic way—releasing these chemicals to help us wake up in the morning, then gradually decreasing the release throughout the day until bedtime. The adrenals work with the hypothalamus and the pituitary gland. This system is called the hypothalamus-pituitary-adrenal axis, often referred to as the HPA axis.

It's important to remember that our body is always trying its best to maintain balance (homeostasis) and protect us from harm! This system has been in place for thousands of years. It's easy to imagine that what our body perceives as stress and danger in the modern world is quite different from what our hunter-gatherer ancestors dealt with! While we might feel stressed about our boss's expectations, homework, or holiday shopping, our ancestors were worried about woolly mammoths and starvation. And yet, our hormone system is the same and so the same responses are triggered, whether it's an e-mail from your angry boss or a bear lurking in the bushes. The adrenals release cortisol and adrenaline to get us ready to fight. Our blood sugar levels go up and our blood goes to our limbs so that we can run for our life. The heart rate goes up to make sure our muscles get plenty of oxygen to run or fight. The beautiful thing about this healthy response to danger is that all these responses quiet right back down once the danger is over—and we recover. Cortisol, known as the stress hormone, is a very useful and good thing to have. However, in our modern life, many of us are in a chronic state of stress and all these responses are happening all the time. Consistently high levels of cortisol over long periods of time is what can lead to other health problems, such as weight gain, depression, sleep problems, and thyroid issues.

Most modern-day chronic diseases and ailments can be linked to lifestyle factors and stress. Adding healthy habits, self-care, and adaptogens may help both prevent and even overcome existing chronic problems.

MOOD

Feeling, atmosphere, attitude, spirit, temperament—*mood* is a broad term all about how we are doing mentally and emotionally. Sometimes we're in a bad mood for no explicable reason. We feel sluggish, uninspired, down on ourselves, and sad. Other times, life feels light and easy. Have you ever considered that your mood could be affected by what you put in your body? By the foods you choose to eat or not to eat? The powerful plants described in this book have the ability to uplift your spirit, get you to relax when you need to, and help you stay calm and avoid reacting as excessively and aggressively to stress. Life happens and there will always be things that are stressful. While you can't always change your environment, you can change how you react!

SLEEP

Hopefully, you have heard that sleep is really important to our health. Like, seriously vital for longevity and well-being. But it's often undervalued. And maybe even worse: when we want to and try to go to sleep, we simply can't! For so many of us, our body is too stressed out, amped up, and excited to go to sleep at night. Stress messes with the body's natural circadian rhythm. If we lived in an area without electricity, we would rise with the sun and rest when the sun had set. Today, most of us are not at all in tune with nature's rhythms and we sit inside with bright lights on, watching electronic screens, even when it's dark outside. Cortisol actually responds to light and dark, when functioning normally. It's natural for cortisol levels to be higher in the morning and then taper off as the day goes on. Stress often causes cortisol to be released in higher doses later in the day, which keeps us amped up and awake at bedtime. Trying to tune in more to nature's rhythm, dim the lights inside, and avoid viewing screens before bed can really help improve our quality of sleep.

If you're someone struggling with getting enough good-quality sleep, you want to know about adaptogens! A restful night's sleep is a birthright and adaptogens and herbs can help your body calm down, release, and relax to get that much-needed sleep. Even though adaptogens don't have the ability to put you to sleep the way a medication could, they can work with your body and help regulate cortisol to help you chill out at night. When your body is more relaxed and balanced, it also has an easier time falling asleep and getting the rest it needs at night.

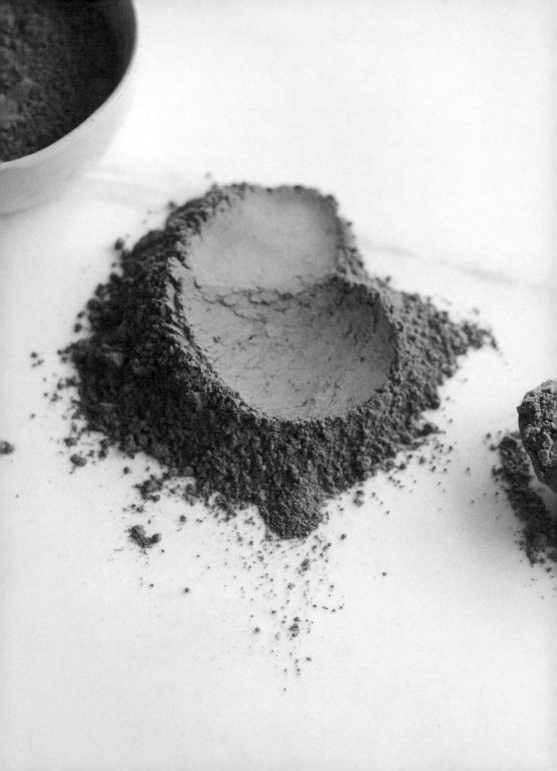

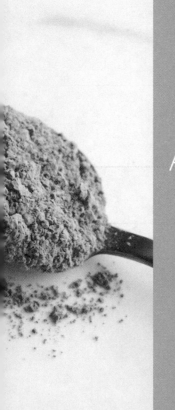

PART TWO.
ADAPTOGENS
AND MUSHROOMS

Adaptogens work slowly and gently. No crashes here! These plants adapt their function according to your body's specific needs. It feels almost magical!

Amla: rejuvenating, digestive support, skin

Ashitaba: concentration, beauty, longevity

Ashwagandha: calming, new-mom support, libido booster

Astragalus: immunity booster, whole body toner, healing

Chaga: strength, resilience, healing

Cordyceps: energy booster, antioxidant, immunity support

Eleuthero: alertness, performance, muscle building

Goji: energy, beauty, longevity

Hawthorn: heart support, protection

He Shou Wu: immunity booster, blood cleanser, youth elixir

Holy basil (tulsi): vitality, mood, soothing

Licorice: belly soother, anti-inflammatory, fatigue fighter

Lion's mane: brain function, concentration, antianxiety

Maca: hormone balance, fertility, mood, libido

Moringa: anxiety relief, digestive support, antioxidant

Mucuna pruriens: mood enhancer, fortifier, motivator

Panax ginseng (Asian ginseng): mental performance, memory, alertness

Pearl: hair, skin, and nails; radiance; bone health

Pine pollen: brain food, immunity support, libido

Reishi: calming, rejuvenating, immunity support

Rhodiola: clarity, strength, performance

Schisandra berry: skin, detox support, nurtures adrenal glands

Sea buckthorn: skin glow and skin health, digestive support

Shatavari: women's adaptogen, hormone harmonizer, fatigue fighter

Turkey tail: gut health, immunity strengthener

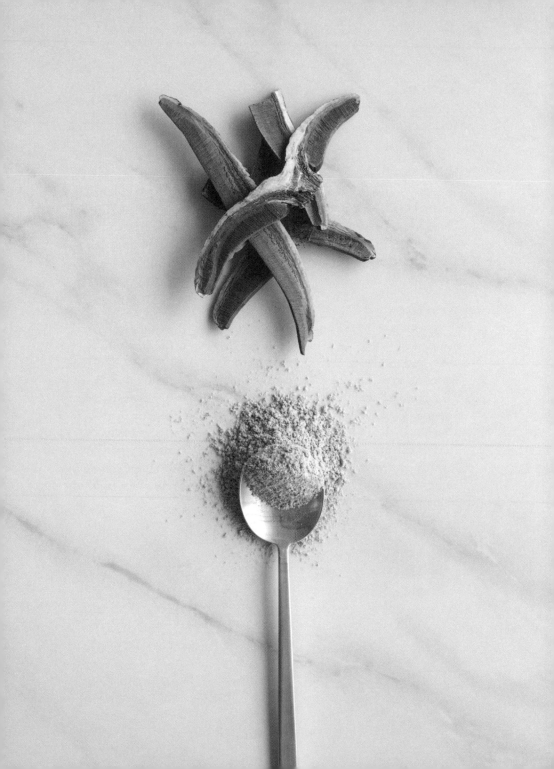

AMLA

REJUVENATING, DIGESTIVE SUPPORT, SKIN

Overview

This ancient Ayurvedic superfood, also known as amalaki or Indian gooseberry, has a sour taste that makes it a good alternative to lemon and lime in cooking. It is a berry and the base of a cherished Ayurvedic superfood called *chyawanprash*, which contains a multitude of herbs, spices, and adaptogens as well as ghee (clarified butter) and honey. Amla's high vitamin C content makes it a great preservative.

Benefits

In addition to being an amazing adaptogen, this berry is packed with antioxidants! It's wonderful for fighting inflammation. It is loaded with vitamin C, which makes it a great supporter of the immune system. Amla is truly wonderful for your skin—your "inner skin," which is the gut and the respiratory tract. It helps support a healthy gut by balancing the delicate intestinal mucus, which is also very important for your body's ability to assimilate the nutrients from your food. It may have a slight laxative effect and is a key ingredient in the popular Ayurvedic blend triphala, which supports cleansing and proper elimination, and is often used to help people with constipation.

Fit for:

- Seasonal changes
- Skin glow seekers
- Tummy troubles
- Back-to-schoolers

Cautions

Amla contains tannins that may potentially interfere with iron absorption and affect certain medication. Therefore, you should wait at least 4 hours between taking amla and any medication.

As always, if you are on any medication, ask your doctor before starting to take any new herbal supplements, and ask your children's pediatrician before giving any supplements to children.

Find it in:
- Blue Latte (page 112)
- Beauty Tonic (page 123)

ASHITABA

CONCENTRATION, BEAUTY, LONGEVITY

Overview

Ashitaba is native to Japan and celebrated there as a beauty food with antiaging benefits. It's a resilient plant that grows along the coast and after you pick its leaves, they will grow back in just 24 hours. Now, that's superpower! We can enjoy its benefits, too, when ingesting it.

Benefits

Ashitaba can help with wound healing, improve digestion, and with memory, focus, and concentration. It's a good plant source of vitamins B_6 and B_{12} as well. These are really key nutrients for energy and well-being. Additionally, ashitaba contains a compound that can help stimulate production of nerve growth hormone in the body, which is important for longevity. It may even give your skin an extra glow!

Fit for:
- Beauty preservers
- Vegans
- Professors and students

Caution
As always, if you are on any medication, ask your doctor before starting to take any new herbal supplements.

Find it in:
- Green Goddess Dressing (page 173)

ASHWAGANDHA

CALMING, NEW-MOM SUPPORT, LIBIDO BOOSTER

Overview
Although it may seem new to us here in the West, ashwagandha has been a go-to medicinal root for thousands of years! In Ayurveda, it has been used to support immunity and is celebrated for its invigorating properties. It's said to give "horselike vigor" to those who use it regularly. Interestingly, ashwagandha's botanical name is *somnifera*, which means "restful sleep"! Not only will this root get you ready to face modern life's stressors, but it will also improve stamina and sexual health.

Benefits
When taken regularly, ashwagandha can help increase vitality, energy, and endurance. It's incredibly versatile and has the ability to regulate the stress hormone cortisol. It can help stabilize your whole hormonal system, also known as the endocrine system, especially the functioning of your thyroid and adrenals. Ashwagandha is the only adaptogen that has been found to have a stimulating effect on the thyroid.

This potent root will help reduce the effect that stress has on your body. If you're feeling run down, overwhelmed, or exhausted, ashwagandha's ability to support normal energy levels and sleep can come in handy. You will likely be able to enjoy your daily life with more energy and vitality. A new mom who is thrown into a whole new reality of sleepless nights, baby cries, and new routines is the perfect candidate for a daily dose of ashwagandha. That feeling of "mom-brain" might benefit from the memory and cognitive support ashwagandha can offer. And, in fact, ashwagandha has long been used in Ayurveda to support new moms with lactation.

Studies have also shown promising results in regard to ashwagandha's ability to strengthen the immune system. It's more common to experience illness when we're stressed, overwhelmed, or exhausted, and ashwagandha can help the body better deal with situations so that we don't end up there in the first place.

Fit for:
- Busy bees
- Run-down overschedulers
- Insomniacs
- Hotheads
- Supermoms (and -dads)

It's actually hard to imagine someone for whom ashwagandha wouldn't be helpful! Anyone with a smartphone that constantly pings with e-mails and calendar reminders or whose day consists of running from one deadline to the next could benefit from its calming effects and its ability to reduce the damaging effects of stress. For people with such common modern-day ailments as high blood pressure, insomnia, or chronic fatigue syndrome, ashwagandha can be a useful tool alongside diet, lifestyle, and prescription medication changes to help get the body back in balance. It also contains a nice dose of antioxidants that help protect the body from damaging oxidative stress. And the high dose of iron found in ashwagandha makes it great for supporting people with anemia.

Cautions

Ashwagandha should be avoided during pregnancy. (In Africa, the herb has traditionally been used to cause miscarriages. While there are no studies confirming this, it's not worth taking the risk when pregnant.)

Ashwagandha may interfere with the effectiveness of any immunosuppressive therapy. People with multiple sclerosis, rheumatoid arthritis, or lupus are usually advised to avoid ashwagandha altogether. Ashwagandha is not recommended if you are taking sedatives or if you have severe gastric irritation or ulcers. Also, this is a nightshade plant, so people who are sensitive to nightshades should be careful.

As always, if you are on any medication, ask your doctor before starting to take any new herbal supplements.

Find it in:

- Beauty Moon Milk (page 113)
- Mayan Hot Chocolate (page 117)
- Coldbrew Iced Latte (page 118)
- Adrenal Tonic (page 122)
- Nightcap Tonic (page 127)
- Warm Winter Tisane (page 130)
- Unbeatable Brownies (page 132)
- Chocolate Milkshake (page 145)
- No-Cook Chocolate Ginger Squares (page 147)
- Spoonfuls (page 151)
- Adaptogenic Nut-Granola (page 163)
- Adaptogenic Honey (page 180)
- Golden Milk Powder Blend (page 181)

ASTRAGALUS

IMMUNITY BOOSTER, WHOLE BODY TONER, HEALING

Overview

Astragalus is another adaptogen that's been tested through time and traditionally used in Chinese medicine for centuries to help protect the body from disease and support the liver. It's a yellow root originally found in China; today, most astragalus found on the market is cultivated.

Benefits

This adaptogen is many practitioners' absolute favorite. It's very toning and great for both the cardiovascular and nervous systems. It's also beneficial for the digestive and immune system. Basically, it supports function in the whole body! Astragalus can also stimulate telomerase, an enzyme in our body that works to restore damaged DNA and in that way fights signs of aging and improves longevity.

Fit for:

- Immunity support
- Teachers and healers
- Heartachers
- Flu recovery

This is a great adaptogen for anyone in recovery from illness but also, when taken regularly, for anyone looking to support overall health.

Cautions

Astragalus is said to have the ability to make a fever last longer, so it's not recommended while you're feeling under the weather. It also may have properties that could alter how medications affect the body, so be absolutely sure to consult a qualified physician before taking astragalus if you are on any medication. Astragalus should therefore be avoided by anyone on immunosuppressants or blood thinners. People with diabetes or hypertension need to avoid this herb, as do pregnant and nursing mothers.

As always, if you are on any medication, ask your doctor before starting to take any new herbal supplements.

Find it in:
- Golden Latte (page 115)
- Detox Tonic (page 129)
- Women's Bonbons (page 137)
- Matcha Bliss Balls (page 141)
- Raw Macaroons Four Ways (page 149)
- Spoonfuls (page 151)
- Golden Sunrise Shake (page 165)
- Blue Against Blues (page 168)
- Pumped-Up Bone Broth (page 179)
- Adaptogenic Honey (page 180)

CHAGA

STRENGTH, RESILIENCE, HEALING

Overview

Chaga is a medicinal mushroom with immense power to heal, strengthen, and support the immune system. In the wild, chaga mushrooms grow on birch trees. They're parasitic and grow from the inside of the tree outward. Chaga has been part of traditional folk medicine for ages and is historically found in birch forests in Russia and northern Europe.

Benefits

Chaga stimulates the immune system and is rich in beta-glucans (the carbohydrates, found in the cells of the fungus, which support healthy immune function). It will give the immune system a boost whenever it's slow and sluggish or can slow it down when it is overactive (as is the case with allergies).

Chaga is also loaded with nutrients and antioxidants. It can help fight fatigue and give you a little boost when you need to get a job done. This makes it a great substitute for coffee and a perfect travel companion, helping you have energy and immunity while away from your usual routine.

Fit for:
- Travelers
- Immunity support
- Anxiety reduction

Caution

As always, if you are on any medication, ask your doctor before starting to take any new herbal supplements.

Find it in:
- Tahini Shrooms Chocolate Spread (page 153)
- Mushroom Broth (page 177)

CORDYCEPS

ENERGY BOOSTER, ANTIOXIDANT, IMMUNITY SUPPORT

Overview

Cordyceps is a type of fungus that grows in the foothills of the Himalayas in Bhutan and Nepal. Collected and traded as early as the Tang dynasty (AD 618 to 907), this medicinal food has long been central to the Tibetan economy! It is used in Chinese medicine and is considered one of the rarest and most valuable herbs. Overharvesting is an issue, so the kind we find on the market in the West today is (and should be) cultivated.

Benefits

Cordyceps has many amazing benefits. It's known to support the endocrine system (a.k.a. your hormonal system) and help you stay balanced during times of stress. It's also great at supporting endurance (both the physical and mental kind!) and the immune system overall. Studies have shown that cordyceps may have a positive effect on blood sugar. Other research has demonstrated improved athletic performance and improved lactate clearance with use of cordyceps—so, if you're looking to up your gym game or attempt a triathlon, you might want to become friendly with cordyceps! This fungus is a celebrated aphrodisiac and said to help improve overall sexual energy. Because it can also help you focus, it can be a helpful tool for students, chess players, and hard workers of any kind.

Fit for:
- Endurance
- The traveler
- Sexual energy
- Endocrine support
- Immunity support

Cautions

There is such a thing as too much of a good thing. Excessive amounts of cordyceps might end up weakening your immune system instead of supporting it.

As always, if you are on any medication, ask your doctor before starting to take any new herbal supplements.

Find it in:
- Meaningful Matcha (page 103)
- Tahini Shrooms Chocolate Spread (page 153)
- Matcha Milkshake (page 164)
- Carrot Ginger Dressing (page 175)
- Mushroom Broth (page 177)

ELEUTHERO

ALERTNESS, PERFORMANCE, MUSCLE BUILDING

Overview

Also known as Siberian ginseng, eleuthero is a root and was the first plant to be classified as an adaptogen. It grows in Siberia as well as northern China, Korea, and Japan. Traditionally, in China, eleuthero was used to make wine to help people recover from low energy.

Benefits

In Chinese medicine, this energy booster has been used to invigorate and support sexual function. Studies have found that this root helped protect people from getting sick by strengthening the immune system. Eleuthero has also been shown to increase the stamina and performance of athletes, which means it's great for anyone who exercises a lot and wants to both perform better and avoid burnout. Improved mental alertness has also been reported with regular use of eleuthero. Because of all those amazing benefits, it's a great supporting adaptogen for those who burn the midnight oil, work the night shift, or just like to play hard.

Fit for:
- Vitality
- Cold and flu busting
- People over 40 looking to increase stamina

Cautions

It's generally recommended to take eleuthero periodically, and not all the time. Ideally, take it for one month and then take two months off.

Because it can boost energy, eleuthero traditionally benefits people over the age of 40 whose metabolisms may be already slowing down.

This adaptogen is usually not recommended for those with high blood pressure. As always, if you are on any medication, ask your doctor before starting to take any new herbal supplements.

Find it in:
- Warm Winter Tisane (page 130)

GOJI

ENERGY, BEAUTY, LONGEVITY

Overview

Goji is native to China and is also known as *Lycium* or Chinese wolfberry. The antioxidant-packed, bright red berries are delicious to eat on their own, as you would raisins, and are used in cooking as well. In dried and powdered form, goji berry can be added easily to smoothies and other prepared dishes.

Benefits

Goji berries are high in carotenoids and flavonoids (antioxidants), which are great for eye health. These berries are also rich in vitamin C and contain all nine of the essential amino acids, making this a true, nutrient-dense superfood! Traditionally goji was used to support eye health and night vision. The berries provide a great energy boost, and their nutrient profile supports vitality and beauty.

Fit for:
- Hikers
- Busy bees
- Beauties

Cautions

Goji berries belong to the nightshade family. If you're sensitive to other nightshades, you might want to avoid goji, too.

People on warfarin, and people taking certain medications for diabetes and blood pressure problems, should not consume goji berries. As always, if you are on any medication, ask your doctor before starting to take any new herbal supplements.

Find it in:
- Quencher (page 125)
- Chocolate Bark (page 133)
- Energy Bars (page 143)
- Raw Macaroons Four Ways (page 149)
- Overnight Chia Oats (page 161)

HAWTHORN

HEART SUPPORT, PROTECTION

Overview

This plant has a special place in folklore and myths. For example, it was the gateway to the faerie world in Celtic folklore, and in ancient Greece, it was used in marriage and birth ceremonies. Hawthorn was also the crown of thorns Jesus wore. Clearly, it's a plant that humans have always seen as meaningful, powerful, and symbolic.

Benefits

In Chinese medicine, hawthorn is considered regenerative for the heart. Traditionally, it was used for depression, anxiety, and to help improve focus, as well as as a digestive tonic. More recent studies have shown that it may in fact have many heart-supportive benefits, including prevention of angina and lowering blood pressure. It's also a great overall anti-inflammatory that will help support optimal health and is packed with antioxidants that protect your body. In addition, hawthorn has been known to offer relief for symptoms of menopause!

Fit for:

- Heart health/heart healing
- Anti-inflammatory support

Cautions

Hawthorn is not recommended while pregnant *or* nursing, but generally considered very safe, even for children. As a supplement, it's recommended for short-term use only.

As always, if you are on any medication, ask your doctor before starting to take any new herbal supplements.

Find it in:

- Pink Latte (page 111)
- Heart Tonic (page 128)
- Unicorn Bowl (page 158)

HE SHOU WU

IMMUNITY BOOSTER, BLOOD CLEANSER, YOUTH ELIXIR

Overview

Ths longevity-boosting root got its name from the man who discovered it. "He Shou Wu" means "black-haired mister." He claimed the root restored his gray hair back to black and gave him the ability to father a child after years of not being able to. The root is also used in Korea, Japan, and Vietnam for slightly different challenges.

Benefits

He Shou Wu is still used today for hair that is graying prematurely, perhaps due to its high zinc level and/or the harmonizing effect it has on the hormonal system. It has been found to stimulate the body to produce longevity-promoting antioxidants. Regular use will help encourage proper liver and gallbladder function. Additionally, like most adaptogens, it supports the immune system. It's also known to calm the nervous system, making it a great herb for busy people. Studies have found it increased the life span of some animals, so one can only hope that translates to humans, too!

On a different note, this adaptogen is traditionally seen as a spirit tonic. It may help bring out your inner creativity and make you feel more receptive and intuitive.

Fit for:

- Graying hair
- The artist
- Spirit seekers
- Meditators

Cautions

Very large doses of He Shou Wu may cause diarrhea. If you are taking statins or any other medication, consult a physician before you start to take He Shou Wu.

As always, if you are on any medication, ask your doctor before starting to take any new herbal supplements.

Find it in:
- Beauty Moon Milk (page 113)
- Women's Bonbons (page 137)
- Chocolate Milkshake (page 145)
- Spoonfuls (page 151)

58

HOLY BASIL (TULSI)

VITALITY, MOOD, SOOTHING

Overview

Holy basil, a.k.a. tulsi, is a superherb with a sacred status. It's believed to be the embodiment of Lakshmi—the Hindu goddess of wealth, love, and prosperity. It's grown in most gardens and courtyards in India and used in prayer and meditation. In Chinese medicine, it is also seen as an herb that nourishes the *shen* (spirit). The leaves of the plant are used for therapeutic purposes, and you could most likely grow holy basil in your own garden!

Benefits

Holy basil supports both the immune and the digestive systems. It can help lower cortisol levels in the body and prevent you from getting stressed out. Because it supports clear breathing, holy basil is also a powerful antioxidant and has been found to be helpful for people with asthma and allergies. It's even possible that it can help lower blood sugar levels. Holy basil can help your body maintain a healthy weight. It's a powerful anti-inflammatory, too, and one of the few adaptogens with antimicrobial effects. It's a great adaptogen to take in the evening to help you unwind from the day and calm down before sleep. And, unlike many other adaptogens that have a more cumulative effect, you may feel calm instantly after consuming holy basil.

Traditionally it's been used to balance the chakras (the energy centers in the body) and can help bring you harmony and balance.

If you're looking for some mental clarity and heightened awareness, add holy basil to your rotation.

Fit for:
- The diabetic
- The asthmatic and seasonal sneezer
- The meditator, yogi, and spirit seeker
- Unwinding

Cautions
Holy basil is a mild diuretic. It is also found to decrease fertility in men.

As always, if you are on any medication, ask your doctor before starting to take any new herbal supplements.

Find it in:
- Warm Winter Tisane (page 130)

LICORICE

BELLY SOOTHER, ANTI-INFLAMMATORY, FATIGUE FIGHTER

Overview
Licorice is the most common herb in Chinese medicine and is often used in small amounts alongside other herbs. Its sweet taste helps make other herbs more palatable, too! It's also traditionally been used as both a food and medicine in the Middle East to benefit people with dry coughs and respiratory issues—and it is still used for those same issues today.

Benefits
Licorice is used in many herbal blends as a harmonizer. On its own, it's beneficial for stomach issues, such as bloating and irri-

table bowel syndrome (IBS). Many practitioners also give a form of this to people dealing with leaky gut, as it's both soothing and anti-inflammatory! It's used to support adrenal fatigue as well, and for those feeling exhausted all the time.

Fit for:
- IBS, inflammatory bowel disease (IBD), and other digestive symptoms
- Low energy and fatigue

Caution
Licorice can have a number of harmful effects when taken for a prolonged period of time. For starters, it should not be used by pregnant women. It should be avoided by anyone with high blood pressure/hypertension, heart disease, edema, low blood potassium, or a liver disorder. Ingesting large doses of licorice may cause excess retention of sodium and excretion of potassium; when you consume licorice powder or blends containing licorice powder, do not exceed the dose recommended on the package.

As always, if you are on any medication, ask your doctor before starting to take any new herbal supplements.

LION'S MANE

BRAIN FUNCTION, CONCENTRATION, ANTIANXIETY

Overview
This edible mushroom looks like a hairy mane, as its name reflects (or some might say it looks like a cheerleader's pom-pom), and has been found to have some amazing benefits. Traditionally, lion's mane was used in Chinese medicine and in Japan, and at different times in history, it was reserved for only the royals. It is celebrated by Buddhist monks as an amazing source of nutrients. It's still unclear whether lion's mane should be considered an adaptogen or

not, as the definition of *adaptogen* is itself somewhat fluid and there is no authority that actually decides which herbs are adaptogens and which are not. However, this is, without a doubt, a powerful supermushroom well worth knowing about and including alongside the other super powders in this book.

Benefits

Lion's mane contains something called nerve growth factors, which actually can help regenerate and protect brain tissue. This is exciting in this day and age, when so many people suffer from brain-degenerative diseases, such as Alzheimer's and Parkinson's. It is loaded with antioxidants and has anti-inflammatory benefits, too. Lion's mane has even been found to lower depression and anxiety. It contains a very beneficial beta-glucan (a polysaccharide, a.k.a. a complex carbohydrate) that we know is beneficial for heart health and a healthy immune response. It's no wonder that this mushroom is generating a lot of interest among medical researchers.

Fit for:

· Brain support and health

· Memory and concentration

· Anxiety and depression

· Immunity support

Caution

As always, if you are on any medication, ask your doctor before starting to take any new herbal supplements.

Find it in:

· Tahini Shrooms Chocolate Spread (page 153)

· Carrot Ginger Dressing (page 175)

· Mushroom Broth (page 177)

MACA

HORMONE BALANCE, FERTILITY, MOOD, LIBIDO

Overview

Maca is a starchy tuber from the Andes Mountains in South America. This stubborn root seems to thrive in the most challenging environments. Traditionally, in Peru, maca was eaten as a food, although today it's most often sold in powder form. It has a pleasant malty taste reminiscent of vanilla or butterscotch, making it a great addition to smoothies and lattes.

Benefits

Maca has a great reputation as an aphrodisiac and has been shown in several studies to have a positive effect on libido. It's a known hormone supporter and a trusted friend of menopausal women. It's even believed to have some positive effects on male fertility by increasing sperm count. It's also a wonderful energy and endurance booster. According to legend, Incan warriors used to consume maca before heading into battle. These days, many head into "battle" on a daily basis, so maca can be a great tool for keeping fit for a fight! Additionally, maca can be a nice mood enhancer when you're feeling a bit bogged down. It has been consumed medicinally in Peru for thousands of years, and has anxiety-reducing and antidepressant effects.

It's quite nutritious, too! Maca is a decent source of potassium, magnesium, calcium, iron, and iodine. Iodine is an important nutrient that can be hard to find! Every 2 teaspoons (10 grams) of maca powder contains about 0.052 mg of iodine, which is about 35 percent of the recommended daily allowance based on the 0.150 mg daily guideline. Maca's vitamin C content makes it a great immunity booster! In addition, the root is rich in amino acids that are the building blocks for hormones. This nourishing and building food can help boost energy, sex drive, and stamina, and lift your mood. Maca comes in red, black, and cream. Red is best for women, black is best for men, and cream can be used by all.

Fit for:

- Baby-makers
- Menopause
- Mood lifting
- Modern world warriors

Cautions

Maca belongs to the cruciferous vegetable family and contains high levels of glucosinolates (sulfur-containing compounds that, when consumed in large amounts, can have negative effects on the thyroid). So if you have a thyroid condition, you may want to avoid eating larger amounts of these foods in their raw state. If you're buying maca as a powder supplement, look for gelatinized maca that has been boiled and pressurized to remove the starch before turning it into a powder. It's not actually gelatinous and blends easily into foods and drinks.

Maca can get moldy during the drying process of the root, and if this happens, the final product may contain aflatoxin, a known carcinogen. Therefore, always buy high-end maca from trusted brands! Check out the Maca Team if you're looking for a good-quality source of gelatinized maca.

As always, if you are on any medication, ask your doctor before starting to take any new herbal supplements.

Find it in:

- Beauty Chai (page 101)
- Tahini Maca Latte (page 109)
- Mayan Hot Chocolate (page 117)
- Unbeatable Brownies (page 132)
- Energy Bars (page 143)
- Raw Macaroons Four Ways (page 149)

MORINGA

ANXIETY RELIEF, DIGESTIVE SUPPORT, ANTIOXIDANT

Overview

The moringa tree is native to Africa and the Himalayas in Asia. Its leaves can be dried and turned into a convenient powder. These leaves are incredibly nutrient-dense, with a spinach flavor that works well in smoothies and matcha drinks. Moringa can also be applied topically in oil form. The tree itself is very fast growing and can grow in even dry and nutrient-poor soil—it's even used in reforestation efforts and for soil fertilization. Moringa has been utilized in Ayurvedic medicine for 4,000 years!

Benefits

Moringa contains a good amount of protein and is an excellent source of iron and vitamins A, B_6, and C, as well as antioxidants! The plant has also been known to lower cholesterol and reduce inflammation. In addition, it contains an acid that has been found to help control blood sugar levels, which gives moringa both hormone-balancing and antidiabetic benefits. It may help support digestion, as it contains both fiber and calcium that can boost digestive enzyme production. Tryptophan, an amino acid the body needs to make serotonin, is found in moringa, too, making this super powder a great mood stabilizer!

Your skin will benefit from the dose of vitamins A and E found in moringa, and its incredibly high antioxidant content may help prevent damage to the skin and inhibit those early signs of aging.

Fit for:
- Breastfeeding mamas
- Wellness seekers
- Skin concerns

Caution

When you buy moringa, it should be labeled as "moringa leaf powder." Moringa root may be toxic and should not be consumed.

As always, if you are on any medication, ask your doctor before starting to take any new herbal supplements.

Find it in:
- Meaningful Matcha (page 103)
- Raw Macaroons Four Ways (page 149)
- Green Goddess Dressing (page 173)

MUCUNA PRURIENS

MOOD ENHANCER, FORTIFIER, MOTIVATOR

Overview

Mucuna pruriens is a climbing vine native to Africa and Asia. A legume, it is often called the velvet bean because of its hairy and leathery pods. Many indigenous cultures eat the beans as a good source of protein and because of its uplifting mood benefits. While the whole plant can be used, the seeds inside the pods are what are harvested and turned into a super powder for our consumption. It's also been used in Ayurvedic medicine for centuries and is believed to be a powerful aphrodisiac and a pain reliever.

Benefits

Mucuna pruriens is a psychoactive (as is coffee), but unlike coffee, it is nonaddictive. Its seed contains a compound called L-dopa, which is a precursor of the neurotransmitter dopamine, a chemical in the brain that affects emotions, movements, and sensations of pleasure and pain; it also stimulates the reward center in the brain. With increased dopamine signaling comes a delicious mood boost. So, basically, *Mucuna pruriens* works as a natural mood enhancer! In addition, because it contains L-dopa, it is a natural aphrodisiac, helping increase pleasure. This remarkable plant shares some of the same properties, in trace amounts, as ayahuasca and tobacco! You may very possibly experience more vivid dreams and deeper sleep after taking it. It's also celebrated as a spiritual and consciousness-enhancing plant. When taking *Mucuna pruriens*, you may experience a decrease in stress (especially of the emotional kind), clarity, and an increase in overall well-being.

The L-dopa stimulates the pituitary gland to produce human growth hormone, which helps improve muscle growth and strength. It's also been shown to help lower levels of prolactin, which in turn can reduce menstrual discomfort and the weight gain that can come with it, as well as improve fertility in men.

Mucuna pruriens has been widely studied in recent years because L-dopa is a substance used as a treatment for Parkinson's disease.

Fit for:
- Psychological/emotional stress
- Anxiety and depression
- Wellness junkies

Cautions

Mucuna pruriens is best taken separately from food, if possible, and is not recommended for frequent consumption. One option is to do a couple of weeks on and then a week off.

As always, if you are on any medication, ask your doctor before starting to take any new herbal supplements.

Find it in:
- Meaningful Matcha (page 103)
- Good Mood Matcha (page 107)
- Beauty Moon Milk (page 113)

- Mayan Hot Chocolate (page 117)
- Coldbrew Iced Latte (page 118)
- Blue Lagoon Lemonade (page 126)
- No-Cook Chocolate Ginger Squares (page 147)
- Spoonfuls (page 151)
- Adaptogenic Honey (page 180)

PANAX GINSENG (ASIAN GINSENG)

MENTAL PERFORMANCE, MEMORY, ALERTNESS

Overview

This Asian herb is one of the most celebrated and studied plants out there. Traditionally, it has been used as a longevity tonic. Panax ginseng used to grow in the mountainous forests of China and Korea, but overharvesting and mismanagement have led to the loss of wild ginseng. All Asian ginseng on the market today is cultivated.

Benefits

Panax ginseng is one of the more stimulating adaptogens, and yet it is balancing in its effect. While it may be uplifting for some people (those who may need that boost), it can feel calming to others (who may already be a bit anxious and high-strung). It can even provide a little mood lift when needed!

Ginseng helps oxygenate the body and increases libido in both men and women. Its most celebrated benefit, however, is its effect on brain function. Ginseng has been found to help improve memory, prevent age-related cognitive decline, improve learning speed and retention, and boost alertness.

Ginseng can also help normalize immune function, whether your system is overactive (as is the case with allergies or autoimmunity) or depleted (as is the case with cancer or chronic fatigue).

People who are run down, depleted, fatigued, or dealing with adrenal exhaustion can benefit greatly from ginseng's uplifting and stimulating effect.

Ginseng has been found to have a nice stabilizing effect on blood sugar and is an anti-inflammatory.

Fit for:
- Students
- Night shift workers
- The worn-out, tired, and depleted

Caution
Ginseng may make symptoms worse for people who experience insomnia, hypertension, or who are generally anxious. As always, if you are on any medication, ask your doctor before starting to take any new herbal supplements.

PEARL

HAIR, SKIN, AND NAILS; RADIANCE; BONE HEALTH

Overview
Pearl powder is basically ground up freshwater pearls. It's a legendary beauty food and the one and only Cleopatra was a fan. Ancient peoples in India, Egypt, and some indigenous cultures in South and Central America have ingested it.

Benefits
The beauty benefits of pearl come from its ability to stimulate collagen production, helping the skin stay youthful, plump, and glowing. It may help regenerate new skin cells and improve the radiance of the skin. Pearl is rich in calcium and other minerals that are strengthening to hair, skin, and nails; it promotes healing as well. Its calcium is beneficial for bone health and bone density. Pearl

also has anti-inflammatory and antioxidant properties. While the powder does wonders from the inside out, it works great topically, too. You can add it to a mask, serum, or cream!

Fit for:
- Skin glow and strength
- Strong bones, nails, and hair

Cautions

Make sure to ingest only pearl powder intended for internal use and don't consume more than the recommended dose, since larger amounts can make you very ill.

As always, if you are on any medication, ask your doctor before starting to take any new herbal supplements.

Find it in:
- Beauty Chai (page 101)
- Tahini Maca Latte (page 109)
- Coldbrew Iced Latte (page 118)
- Beauty Tonic (page 123)
- Women's Bonbons (page 137)
- Unicorn Bowl (page 158)
- Blue Against Blues (page 168)
- Raspberry Chia Jam (page 170)

PINE POLLEN

BRAIN FOOD, IMMUNITY SUPPORT, LIBIDO

Overview

This adaptogenic powder is exactly what you think it is—the pollen of a pine tree! Pollen contains the life force and fundamental nutrients for a new life—in this case, it's the life of a new giant tree.

And thus, pine pollen is a nutrient-dense, potent, and healing super powder! It has been used in Chinese medicine for thousands of years and is rapidly gaining popularity in the West. The pollen is usually harvested from the pine cones of wild trees in their natural habitat during their pollination season.

Benefits

Pine pollen has both antiviral and anti-inflammatory properties and is rich in vitamins, minerals, and amino acids. It even contains vitamin D_3, which is hard to find in a food source. Because this is a truly wild food, it's also believed to help connect us to nature and our essence on a spiritual level. Pine pollen is celebrated as a rejuvenation tonic. It can have a great balancing effect on the endocrine system. It is the only known plant containing the hormone DHEA—a precursor to testosterone, estrogen, and progesterone. In the human body, DHEA is produced by the adrenals—those very same glands that tend to get overworked in our very busy lives! There's no wonder a daily dose of pine pollen is helping so many people feel better. DHEA, at healthy levels, will increase libido, boost mood and immunity, and pump up the sex drive.

Pine pollen is, in fact, the only food from the natural world that can actually work like a natural testosterone replacement therapy, meaning it may boost your body's testosterone levels. And yes, while testosterone is the male hormone, women need some testosterone, too. As we get older, testosterone production in our body may decrease, and in those cases the pine pollen boost may offer great support.

Note that to get the androgen benefit of pine pollen, it should be absorbed through the mucous membrane in the mouth into the bloodstream and not the stomach. The harsh conditions of the stomach can destroy those hormones. An easy way to achieve absorption can be to dissolve the powder in a little water and just hold it under your tongue for a few seconds before swallowing. And, even if you simply add the pine pollen powder to a recipe and swallow it down, you'll still get all the benefits of its nutrients!

Fit for:

- Aphrodisiac use
- Metabolism boosting
- Endocrine system rejuvenation
- Hormone balancing

Cautions

Yes—this is a tree pollen, so if you have allergies and notice those symptoms flaring up after taking pine pollen, be sure to check with your doctor: you might need to take a lower dose or avoid it altogether. In general, make sure to stick to recommended or lower doses of pine pollen.

As always, if you are on any medication, ask your doctor before starting to take any new herbal supplements.

Find it in:

- Blue Latte (page 112)
- Chocolate Bark (page 133)
- Raw Macaroons Four Ways (page 149)
- Blue Against Blues (page 168)

REISHI

CALMING, REJUVENATING, IMMUNITY SUPPORT

Overview

Meet the most studied plant on earth! Reishi is a mushroom, known as the queen healer mushroom, and its Chinese name translates to "spirit plant," as it's celebrated as a plant that nourishes the spirit. It was discovered in China in 396 BC and emperors used reishi tonic as part of their quest for immortality. More recent studies have found that reishi indeed contains several compounds that may support longevity. There are many varieties, ranging from red, purple, blue-green, black, and white. The red and purple varieties are seen as superior.

Benefits
There are very few things that reishi doesn't support in the body. It's an overall strengthening and balancing supermushroom! It can help relax the nervous system to calm your body and mind. And because it's packed with antioxidants, it helps protect your skin as well as your cells' DNA and mitochondria (energy centers) from getting damaged by oxidation and stress. Reishi has even been found to stimulate activity in brain neurons. It strengthens the liver, aids in detoxification, and boosts the immune system overall. Reishi may also help support the hormone system and improve sleep. It's one of the adaptogens that are good to consume right before bed as it helps calm the nervous system and supports good-quality sleep! Ganoderic acid, found in reishi, can help inhibit histamine release and improve the use of oxygen. That means it may help alleviate those very annoying seasonal allergies. In addition, reishi may improve your cardiovascular function and it is a great overall preventative superfood. Reishi's antioxidants, along with its anti-inflammatory properties, make it a potential life extender. Studies done on reishi in relation to cancer have found that, in addition to providing immunity support, it may have some antitumor activity.

Fit for:
- The high-strung and stressed-out
- Immunity support
- Sleep
- Seasonal allergies

Cautions
Avoid if you have mushroom allergies. Use caution with reishi if on any blood-thinning medications.

As always, if you are on any medication, ask your doctor before starting to take any new herbal supplements.

Find it in:
- Good Mood Matcha (page 107)
- Golden Latte (page 115)
- Reishi Hot Chocolate (page 116)
- Oranges & Cream (page 124)
- Matcha Bliss Balls (page 141)
- Tahini Shrooms Chocolate Spread (page 153)
- Green Popcorn (page 155)
- Unicorn Bowl (page 158)
- Matcha Milkshake (page 164)
- Carrot Ginger Dressing (page 175)
- Mushroom Broth (page 177)
- Pumped-Up Bone Broth (page 179)

RHODIOLA

CLARITY, STRENGTH, PERFORMANCE

Overview
This tough arctic plant grows wild in Siberia, Tibet, Canada, and Scandinavia and has been used by cultures in these regions for centuries. In fact, the Vikings used rhodiola to enhance physical and mental endurance. And in Siberia, rhodiola was consumed regularly in the coldest months to help prevent getting sick. This is a plant that thrives in conditions that hardly any other plants can survive, and that kind of strength and resilience can be of great benefit to us.

Benefits
This is, without a doubt, the athlete's best friend. Rhodiola can improve physical performance and is generally strengthening.

Athletes in extreme training can use rhodiola both to boost their performance and ease their recovery.

Like all adaptogens, it helps with stress management, and rhodiola actually lowers cortisol (stress hormone) secretion.

Rhodiola is also balancing, in that it can simultaneously be calming emotionally and cognitively stimulating—depending on where your body's needs are. It can help you stay alert and improve memory and mental clarity—which means it might be helpful before a big exam or important work presentation. Additionally, it improves your brain's oxygen-absorbing abilities and increases serotonin, a neurotransmitter that, among other things, affects sleep, mood, and appetite. Rhodiola can have blood sugar–regulating effects, helping you stay well balanced. It contains antioxidants that help protect your body from damage, and has both aphrodisiac and antidepressive benefits. Rhodiola has been found to reduce fatigue symptoms and has been helpful in treating and preventing immunity depletion.

Fit for:

- The tired and run down
- Blood sugar support
- Athletes and performers
- Commuters and travelers
- Anxiety or depression

Cautions

Rhodiola may cause insomnia in some people.

As always, if you are on any medication, ask your doctor before starting to take any new herbal supplements.

Find it in:

- Beauty Chai (page 101)
- Quencher (page 125)

- Detox Tonic (page 129)
- Warm Winter Tisane (page 130)
- Chocolate Bark (page 133)
- Adaptogenic Honey (page 180)

SCHISANDRA BERRY

SKIN, DETOX SUPPORT, NURTURES ADRENAL GLANDS

Overview
Schisandra is also known as magnolia vine and is a climbing plant with pink leaves and red berries. The berries are harvested and dried for medicinal use. The plant is native to China and Russia and parts of Korea. In Chinese, its name means "fruit of the five flavors" and it was celebrated for its ability to preserve youth and beauty. Russian hunters used it as a fatigue-fighting tea and Chinese medicine uses it to balance yin and yang. This is another plant that people seem to disagree about whether it belongs to the adaptogen group or not; however, with its high antioxidant content, balancing effect, and immunity-supporting ability, I think it fits well enough here!

Benefits
This great berry has an overall balancing effect on the endocrine system. We tend to get sick when experiencing a particularly stressful time, and Schisandra helps support this part of the immune system! The berries are also a great source of vitamin C—another important nutrient for immunity. It's seen as a blood nourisher and is found to have a stabilizing effect on blood pressure, too. It will either help raise or lower it, depending on what's needed in each person. Schisandra is generally calming and can help relieve anxiety while boosting work performance.

Fit for:
- Anxiety
- Immunity support
- Skin health
- Endurance and strength

Cautions

Some studies have found that Schisandra may increase stomach acids, which can be helpful in some people, but a problem for others. If you have any history of ulcers or gastritis or just overall high stomach acid, you should not take Schisandra.

Not for use during pregnancy or breastfeeding, unless your physician says it's okay.

As always, if you are on any medication, ask your doctor before starting to take any new herbal supplements.

Find it in:
- Quencher (page 125)
- Chocolate Milkshake (page 145)
- Unicorn Bowl (page 158)
- Love the Skin You're In (page 169)

SEA BUCKTHORN

SKIN GLOW AND SKIN HEALTH, DIGESTIVE SUPPORT

Overview

This wonder-berry is also known as "holy fruit." It contains all of the omega acids, including the very rare, skin-loving omega-7. It's mostly found in Europe and Asia. Its small orange berries get utilized for oils and powders. Legend has it that ancient Greeks gave sea buckthorn to their racehorses, which gave the plant its botanical name *Hippophae*, meaning "shiny horse."

Benefits

This little orange berry is packed with minerals, vitamins A and E, and antioxidants as well as those aforementioned omegas. It's often used for improving skin health and such conditions as psoriasis, but also is generally antiaging and nourishes the skin. It can help strengthen the immune and digestive systems and may encourage weight loss. And, traditionally, sea buckthorn has been used to treat colds and flu.

Fit for:

- Skin health
- Longevity
- Gut health

Cautions

May have blood pressure–lowering effects and may slow blood clotting.

As always, if you are on any medication, ask your doctor before starting to take any new herbal supplements.

Find it in:

- Overnight Chia Oats (page 161)
- Love the Skin You're In (page 169)
- Raspberry Chia Jam (page 170)

SHATAVARI

WOMEN'S ADAPTOGEN, HORMONE HARMONIZER, FATIGUE FIGHTER

Overview

The word *shatavari* translates to "she who has hundreds of husbands." This adaptogen is an ancient aphrodisiac and fertility booster. The plant is in the lily family and native to India and Southeast Asia as well as Australia and Africa. In the Ayurvedic apothecary, shatavari is probably the most important herb for women's health and is used in several formulas.

Benefits

Shatavari has been used to help rebalance minor hormonal imbalances in women and so it may both help stimulate libido and boost fertility. It actually contains precursors to the hormone progesterone. Herbalists may also use shatavari to ease symptoms in menopausal women. It helps support the adrenal glands and balance production of cortisol and has anti-inflammatory as well as immunity-supporting effects. Shatavari is related to asparagus and, like asparagus, is a diuretic that can help soothe urinary challenges. Nursing moms may find their milk flow increase when taking shatavari. Overall, shatavari can support recovery from fatigue and aid in dealing with stress.

Fit for:

- Fatigue and stress
- Libido
- Irritability
- Menopause and hormone balancing

Cautions

Do not take shatavari if you have a history of estrogen-receptor-positive cancer.

As always, if you are on any medication, ask your doctor before starting to take any new herbal supplements.

TURKEY TAIL

GUT HEALTH, IMMUNITY STRENGTHENER

Overview

Turkey tail is another amazing medicinal mushroom celebrated for centuries by Chinese medicine and in Japan, where they are often called cloud mushrooms. This mushroom grows on dead or fallen trees and stumps and can be found all over the world. The colors and pattern on this fungus resemble a turkey's tail.

Benefits

Turkey tail is an adaptogen with great immune function support. Traditionally turkey tail tea has been used to boost the body's resilience to infection and illness. Its ancient use as an immune system aid has led to a lot of interest among medical researchers. Turkey tail can also be beneficial to those undergoing chemotherapy. This mushroom is a prebiotic, meaning it contains fibers that feed the bacteria in your gut. It supports healthy digestion, decreases bloat, and, supports immunity, as a healthy gut flora is key for immunity! Turkey tail is yet another mushroom containing beta-glucan, a complex carb with immunity-boosting power.

Fit for:

- Flu season
- Disease fighters

Caution

As always, if you are on any medication, ask your doctor before starting to take any new herbal supplements.

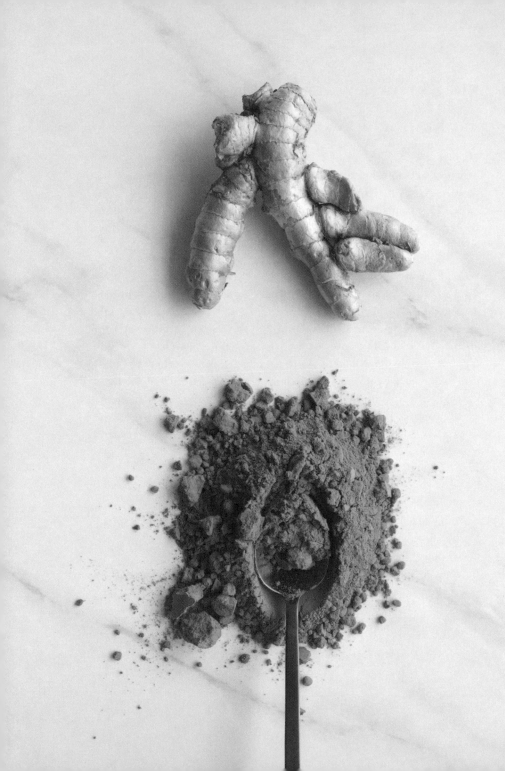

OTHER SUPER POWDERS

These super powders do not act as adaptogens, but have other amazing benefits and are convenient powders that can easily be added to smoothies, tea, coffee, or treats alongside the adaptogens to make these foods provide even more benefits and wellness!

BAOBAB

81

This fruit comes from the African baobab tree, also known as the tree of life. This delicious fruit powder is a great source of vitamin C, antioxidants, and a range of minerals, including magnesium and potassium. The vitamin C helps support collagen production and the antioxidants protect the skin from aging and support that glow-from-within look. Additionally, because baobab contains a lot of fiber (50% of the powder is fiber!), by adding it to sweeter foods, you can slow down your insulin response to those sugars and ensure steady release of energy. The fiber also works as a prebiotic that feeds the good bacteria in your gut, and so baobab can be a great digestive support, too. It's a great natural electrolyte (because of the amount of trace minerals in it) and the taste makes it a perfect fit for smoothies and lemonades.

Find it in:
- Adrenal Tonic (page 122)
- Raspberry Chia Jam (page 170)

BEET

The bright color of beets means they are chock-full of antioxidants. Beets also have anti-inflammatory benefits and are a celebrated heart-supporting food. They contain B vitamins, calcium, and iron. They are known to have a blood-cleansing effect by helping remove toxins and waste from the blood, and support healthy bile flow, which is important for the digestion of fats. Athletes can use beet powder or juice to help with muscle recovery and to build stamina. The natural sweetness of beets makes beet powder a tasty addition to smoothies and lattes.

Find it in:
- Pink Latte (page 111)
- Heart Tonic (page 128)
- Raw Macaroons Four Ways (page 149)

BLUE MAJIK (BLUE SPIRULINA)

Blue Majik is an extract of spirulina, a sea algae, and a potent antioxidant. It has a brilliant blue color and is almost tasteless in small doses, making it both a fun and easy addition to pretty much anything your heart desires! In addition, it is anti-inflammatory and has been shown to inhibit the release of histamines, making it a great food for anyone dealing with allergies. Spirulina is considered a complete protein. It's also a good source of B vitamins, which are important for strength, endurance, and boosting energy levels.

Find it in:
- Blue Latte (page 112)
- Blue Lagoon Lemonade (page 126)
- Unicorn Bowl (page 158)
- Blues Against Blues (page 168)

CACAO POWDER

Cacao is the raw, unprocessed version of what many know as cocoa, and comes from the seedpods of the cacao tree. It's very high in antioxidants (more than wine and blueberries!) and a great protecting food for the body. It does contain some caffeine and therefore can be slightly stimulating. It's also a source of magnesium, among other phytonutrients, which so many of us are deficient in. It might explain why so many women especially crave chocolate. This very craving may also come from cacao's ability to act on our neurotransmitters to help boost our mood and increase the feeling of bliss! Let's eat to that.

Find it in:
- Reishi Hot Chocolate (page 116)
- Mayan Hot Chocolate (page 117)
- Unbeatable Brownies (page 132)
- Chocolate Bark (page 133)
- Women's Bonbons (page 137)
- Your Truffles (page 139)
- Chocolate Milkshake (page 145)
- No-Cook Chocolate Ginger Squares (page 147)
- Raw Macaroons Four Ways (page 149)
- Spoonfuls (page 151)
- Tahini Shrooms Chocolate Spread (page 153)

CHARCOAL/ACTIVATED CHARCOAL

Charcoal has an amazing ability to absorb toxins and help pull them out of the body. Therefore, it may help prevent a hangover; relieve digestive upsets, such as gas and bloating; and overall, help your body detox.

Caution

Avoid taking medications, pills, or vitamins within two hours of consuming charcoal. Charcoal will absorb your pills and may miss the toxins you want removed. For this reason, it's also best to consume it away from any food altogether.

Find it in:
- Charcoal Latte (page 105)
- Detox Tonic (page 129)

CHLORELLA

Chlorella is a single-celled algae and a bright green food rich in chlorophyll and protein. It supports detoxification and contains

B vitamins, which boost energy! Chlorella is an antioxidant that helps protect the cells and eliminate free radicals. It supports the immune system and can help regulate hormones. It's a great super-food to add if you're struggling to eat and drink enough dark, leafy greens. For best absorbability, make sure to buy "cracked cell wall chlorella" so that the nutrients are readily available.

Find it in:
- Green Popcorn (page 155)
- Green Goddess Dressing (page 173)

CINNAMON

Cinnamon's sweet, warming deliciousness is reason enough to consume it on a regular basis. Thankfully, it also contains lots of protective antioxidants and is anti-inflammatory, antibacterial, and immunity boosting!

It has been found to lower blood pressure, and does not actually contain any sugar despite its naturally sweet taste. You'll find this wonderful spice in many recipes in this book!

Caution
It is generally recommended to avoid large amounts of cinnamon if taking blood thinning medication. As always, ask your doctor.

Find it in:
- Beauty Chai (page 101)
- Good Mood Matcha (page 107)
- Tahini Maca Latte (page 109)
- Pink Latte (page 111)
- Golden Latte (page 115)
- Mayan Hot Chocolate (page 117)
- Heart Tonic (page 128)
- Unbeatable Brownies (page 132)
- Women's Bonbons (page 137)

- Matcha Bliss Balls (page 141)
- No-Cook Chocolate Ginger Squares (page 147)
- Raw Macaroons Four Ways (page 149)
- Spoonfuls (page 151)
- Overnight Chia Oats (page 161)
- Adaptogenic Nut-Granola (page 163)
- Golden Sunrise Shake (page 165)
- Golden Milk Powder Blend (page 181)

COLLAGEN PEPTIDES

Collagen is the "glue" that hold our body together and what gives our skin its elasticity. It is what forms connective tissue to help seal and heal the lining of the gut. This protein is made in our body, but the production declines with age. It can be found naturally in such foods as bone broth, but can also be consumed easily as a powder known as collagen peptides. The benefits of continuous use vary, but include stronger hair, skin, and nails; gut healing; reduction in cellulite and stretch marks; joint repair; and detox support. Collagen peptides derived from either seafood or beef are readily available (so this is neither a plant-based nor vegan food).

Find it in:
- Beauty Chai (page 101)
- Good Mood Matcha (page 107)
- Golden Latte (page 115)
- Women's Bonbons (page 137)
- Energy Bars (page 143)
- Adaptogenic Nut-Granola (page 163)
- Matcha Milkshake (page 164)
- Blue Against Blues (page 168)
- Love the Skin You're In (page 169)

MATCHA

Matcha is powdered green tea and is loaded with powerful antioxidants, phytonutrients, and vitamins C and E. It helps boost metabolism and has been shown to be beneficial for weight management and weight loss. It is also energizing and contains caffeine, yet isn't acidic and harsh on your stomach the way coffee may be; it's gentler and tends to cause less jitters in people more sensitive to caffeine. Matcha may also help lower blood sugar and cholesterol. It naturally detoxifies the body, thanks to its chlorophyll content.

Find it in:
- Meaningful Matcha (page 103)
- Good Mood Matcha (page 107)
- Matcha Bliss Balls (page 141)
- Raw Macaroons Four Ways (page 149)
- Matcha Milkshake (page 164)

TURMERIC

Turmeric is the most amazing anti-inflammatory and brightly colored spice, used for centuries especially in India. This pungent and aromatic spice is used both culinarily and medicinally. Turmeric is a root and can be found fresh, juiced, or dried into a powder. It's a kitchen staple in many parts of the world where it is often cooked into soups and curries. This makes sense, since turmeric actually helps break down fat and oil, helping reduce gas and bloating. Traditionally, turmeric has been known as a liver-supporting spice that can boost metabolism and help protect the skin. We now know that curcumin, the active ingredient in turmeric and what gives it the bright color, supports cellular repair, the brain, and the nervous system. Its anti-inflammatory effect can help reduce stiffness and joint pain as well as free-radical cells. Turmeric should be combined with black pepper to enhance absorption (as you will see in the recipes in this book).

Find it in:

SOURCING THE GOOD STUFF

Adaptogens are sold in many different forms. There are liquid tinctures, capsules, powdered individual adaptogens and powdered blends, as well as protein powders, chocolates, and instant coffees and teas with adaptogens added. Since this book is titled *Super Powders*, the focus here will be on the powdered form of these plants. Of course, if you prefer, the capsules can be taken as you would any supplement or vitamin and can be a convenient, easy way to take an adaptogen daily. However, it's worth noting that many adaptogens are better absorbed by the body when taken in combination with a fat.

When buying your adaptogens and other super powders, the source, quality, and purity matter. I would go as far as to say that buying low-quality herbs defeats the purpose and you might as well go without. Look for certified organic and/or foraged in the wild herbal powders. You want to look for pesticide-free products so that you can rest assured that you're really buying what you think you're buying and that the plant source was never treated with chemical pesticides or fertilizers. Organic plants will likely have been grown in a more nutrient-rich soil. You also want to look for a "fair-trade certified" label whenever possible. These are powerful plants that carry energy and life force, so I believe sourcing really matters!

Today, many reputable companies sell adaptogens and the prices can vary greatly. Remember, a little goes a long way, so even though a jar might seem expensive up front, chances are, it will last you several months. Your local herbal shop may also sell many of these powders in bulk, which can be a great way to buy small quantities to test something out before fully committing. You can also buy many of these as dried roots that you can grind into powders, using either a strong blender or a coffee grinder. That is definitely the most cost-effective option!

Always read the label and make sure the only ingredient on the label is the herb(s) you're looking for. You might find that the label only lists the botanical name of the plant. Some blends might add stevia, vanilla, or other natural herbs to add flavor, but beyond that, there shouldn't be anything else listed.

Several online companies sell organic and foraged in the wild adaptogens and super powders. These include Mountain Rose Herbs, Moon Juice, Sun Potion, Moodbeli, and Gaia, and the online health food store Thrive Market has a lot of these brands in stock. Also, if you are having a hard time finding a particular plant in powdered form, you can buy capsules instead—simply break them open and use the powder inside. Many of these companies also make blends that are intended to target specific issues or needs. You may see such words as *calm*, *sleep*, *focus*, or *energy* on the packaging. Trying a blend like that can be a fun and convenient way to approach adaptogens and super powders.

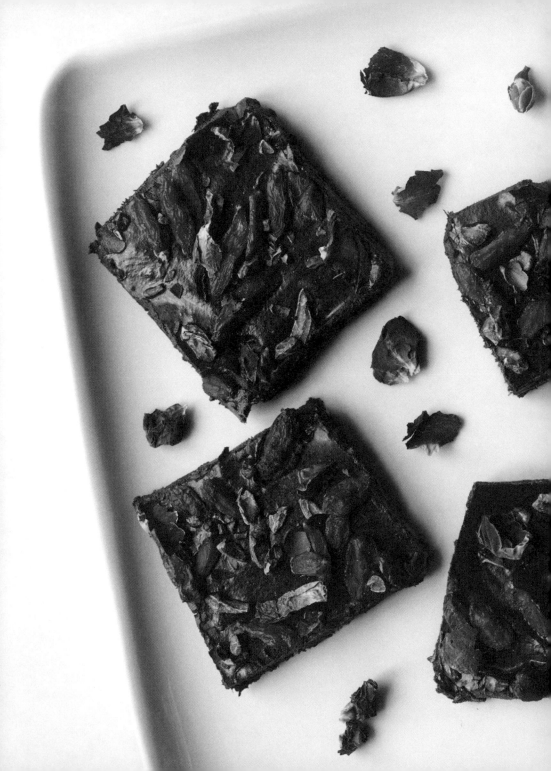

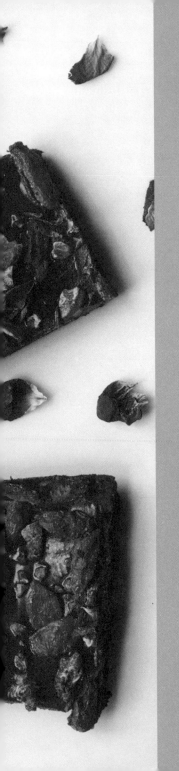

PART THREE.
SUPER POWDER
RECIPES

These recipes are intended to inspire and spark curiosity and experimentation. By no means do you need to follow my exact adaptogen recommendation in each recipe. Feel free to swap my suggestions with your favorite at the moment. If you like things more or less sweet or salty, measure your sweeteners and salt accordingly. You prefer things spicy? Add more ginger or cayenne. Customize these drinks and treats to fit your needs, cravings, and palate. I hope you'll have lots of fun making magic potions and come up with many more yourself.

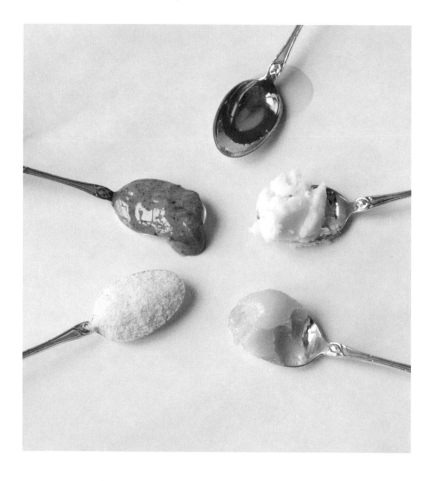

PANTRY

These are the basics you may want to keep handy for making the recipes in this book.

INGREDIENTS

Almonds

Almond butter

Almond flour

Avocado (frozen)

Bananas (frozen)

Black pepper

Blackstrap molasses

Cacao nibs

Cacao powder

Cardamom (ground)

Cashews

Cayenne

Chia seeds

Cinnamon (ground)

Coconut (shredded or
  flakes)

Coconut butter

Coconut meat (frozen)

Coconut oil

Dark chocolate (organic)

Ghee

Ginger (ground)

Goji berries (dried)

Manuka honey

Maple syrup

Medjool dates

Pistachios

Pumpkin puree (canned)

Pumpkin seeds (pepitas)

Raw honey

Rolled oats

Rose water

Sea salt (pink Himalayan
  and regular)

Tahini

Vanilla beans

Vanilla extract

Walnuts

TOOLS

Electric milk frother

Food processor

High-powered blender
(such as a Magic Bullet
or Vitamix)

Matcha whisk

Measuring cups

Measuring spoons

Mixing bowls

Nut milk bag or
cheesecloth

Strainer

LATTES AND DRINKS

These lattes and drinks are not quite the coffee versions you're used to seeing at your local coffee shop. They are nutrient rich, creamy, and truly delicious homemade drinks that will elevate your everyday. Making these at home can quickly become a self-care ritual, as the time it takes to make yourself (or a loved one) a comforting mug of warm milk is such a treat. They come in a rainbow of colors too, from green matcha and golden turmeric lattes to upgraded hot chocolates and mood lifting drinks in hues of blue, pink, and yellow.

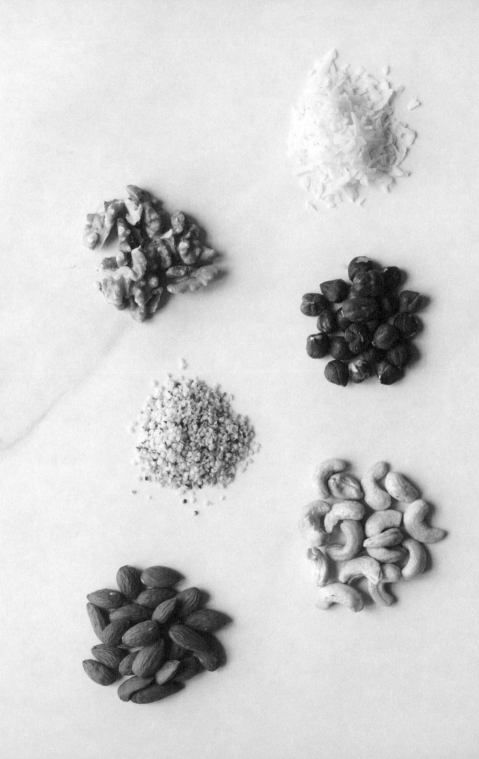

THE BASE

These nut and seed milks are great to have handy for smoothie and latte making. In all the recipes in this book, you can easily replace my suggestion with whichever nut or seed milk you like and have on hand. And there are more nuts and seeds than listed in the recipes here—you can easily use the same methods to make pumpkin seed milk, pecan milk, and so on. Just make sure to start with raw nuts and soak them well for six to eight hours beforehand.

To make a simple adaptogenic latte, warm up one or a combination of the following milks, add your powders of choice, and blend well, using a whisk or milk frother. Add a little raw honey or pure maple syrup, sprinkle with cinnamon powder, and sip slowly. Deep breaths optional.

Pro Tips: For an iced version, simply mix the powders and cold milk, using a whisk or frother, and pour over ice.

For an extra-special version of any nut milk, try soaking your nuts in coconut water!

COCONUT MILK

Coconut milk is absolutely delicious and oh so versatile. From curries to smoothies, coconut milk adds creaminess and a sweet tropical touch. Choose between a sweetened and unsweetened version, depending on your needs. Straining is optional.

Makes 4 servings (about 32 ounces)

3¹⁄₂ cups filtered water (or less if you prefer a thicker result)
2 cups unsweetened shredded coconut
Pinch of sea salt

FOR A SWEET VERSION, ADD:
1 to 2 Medjool dates, pitted
¹⁄₂ teaspoon vanilla extract

1. Place the water, coconut, and salt in a high-speed blender. Add the dates and vanilla, if using.

2. Blend on high speed for 1 to 2 minutes, until the mixture seems smooth.

3. Strain the milk mixture through a nut milk bag suspended over a large bowl. You can also skip this step, if you like! You'll just have a slightly thicker, richer, and more filling nut milk.

4. Store in a lidded container in the fridge for 4 to 5 days. Make sure to shake or stir before pouring, as the milk will separate as it sits.

HEMP MILK

No soaking or straining required for this seed milk, which makes it the easiest of all the milks to make at home.

Makes 4 servings (about 32 ounces)

4 cups filtered water
½ cup raw hemp seeds or hemp hearts
Pinch of sea salt

FOR A SWEET VERSION, ADD:
1 to 2 Medjool dates, pitted
½ teaspoon vanilla extract

1. Place the water, hemp seeds, and salt in a high-speed blender. Add the dates and vanilla, if using.

2. Blend on high speed for 1 to 2 minutes, until the mixture seems smooth.

3. Store in a lidded container in the fridge for 4 to 5 days. Make sure to shake or stir before using, as the milk will separate as it sits.

ALMOND, WALNUT, HAZELNUT, OR CASHEW MILK

These nut milks do require an additional step—soaking the nuts before blending. This allows for the nuts to soften and makes them a lot easier to "milk." It also helps remove some of the phytic acid, an antinutrient that makes the nuts harder to digest.

Makes 4 servings (about 32 ounces)

1 cup raw almonds, walnuts, hazelnuts, or cashews, soaked overnight or for 6 to 8 hours in filtered water
3 to 4 cups filtered water
Pinch of sea salt

FOR A SWEET VERSION, ADD:
2 Medjool dates, pitted, or 2 teaspoons raw honey
1 teaspoon vanilla extract

1. Drain and rinse the soaked nuts.

2. Place the nuts, water, and sea salt in a blender. Add the dates and vanilla, if using.

3. Blend on high speed for 1 minute, or until the liquid looks like milk.

4. Strain the milk mixture through a nut milk bag suspended over a large bowl. Discard the pulp or save it for a different use.

5. Store in a lidded container in the fridge for 2 to 3 days. Make sure to shake or stir before using, as the milk will separate as it sits.

BEAUTY CHAI

Skin, Hormones, Energy

The spices found in traditional chai tea are warming, comforting, and exciting all at once. This version also includes some great skin-benefiting ingredients: pearl for that glowing-from-within skin, collagen to plump and increase elasticity, and maca for hormone balance and energy. The spices are anti-inflammatory and blood sugar balancing, and the heat from the pepper and ginger are great for boosting your digestive fire.

Makes 1 serving

½ cup warm water
1 tablespoon sliced fresh ginger
1 tea bag (black tea, dandelion root, rooibos, or chai blend)
1 cup nut milk (page 100)
4 cardamom pods, smashed
1 cinnamon stick, or ¼ teaspoon ground cinnamon
¼ teaspoon pearl powder
¼ teaspoon maca
¼ teaspoon rhodiola
1 tablespoon collagen peptides
1 teaspoon raw honey

1. Place the warm water and ginger in a small pot and bring to a simmer. Turn down heat, add the tea bag to the water, and let steep. After 5 minutes, remove the ginger and tea bag.

2. Add the nut milk, cardamom pods, and cinnamon stick and gently warm, being careful not to simmer or boil the milk.

3. Strain into a mug and add the adaptogen powders and collagen. Whisk well to combine.

4. Add the raw honey and sip!

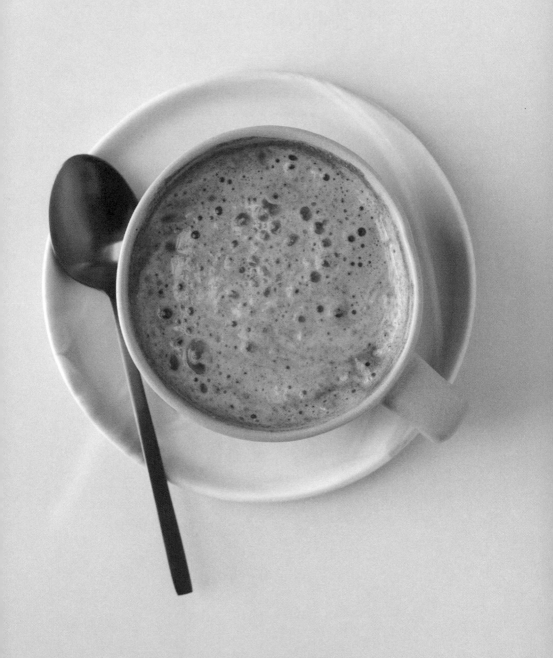

MEANINGFUL MATCHA

Energy, Stamina, Antioxidant Boost

Matcha is a great pick-me-up drink and an excellent, less acidic alternative to coffee! Expect less jitters but lots of focus and energy for the day. It is paired here with moringa, another powerful green powder chock-full of antioxidants, protein, vitamins, and chlorophyll. Make this a warm drink on a cold morning or use cold milk and pour over ice for a refreshing summer drink.

Makes 1 serving

2 teaspoons matcha powder
1 teaspoon cordyceps
1 teaspoon moringa leaf powder
¼ teaspoon Mucuna pruriens
¼ cup warm water
1 cup coconut milk (page 98), warmed
1 teaspoon coconut sugar or coconut nectar

1. Combine the matcha, cordyceps, moringa, *Mucuna pruriens*, and warm water in a mug.

2. Whisk well until all the powders have dissolved and there are no lumps.

3. Add the warm coconut milk and coconut sugar. Stir and sip.

4. If making an iced version, use cold milk instead of warm and pour over ice. If using coconut sugar, you might want to add that in in step 1 to allow it to dissolve in the warm water.

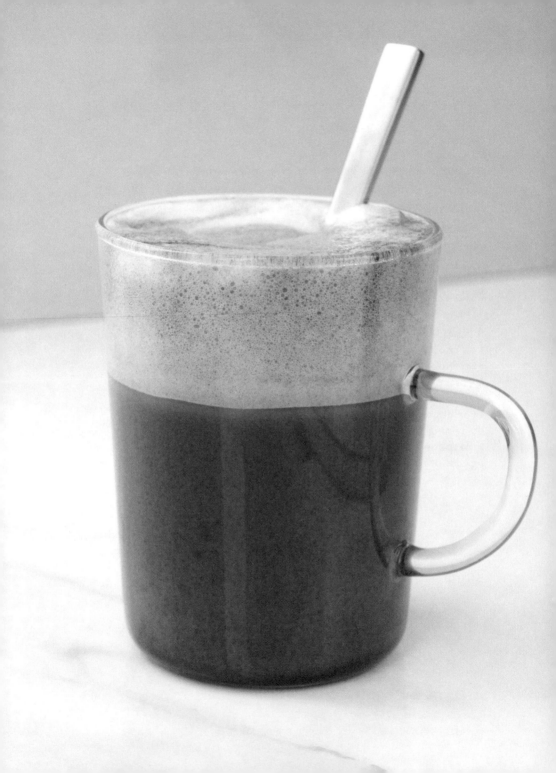

CHARCOAL LATTE

Detox, De-bloat, Hangover Helper

Support detoxification with this spooky-looking latte for the brave. Charcoal helps pull and transport out toxins from your body, making this a good drink the morning after a night of cocktailing. It's also a good remedy for a funny or bloated tummy.

Makes 1 serving

1 cup nut milk (page 100)
1 teaspoon activated charcoal
¼ cup warm (not boiling) water
1 teaspoon vanilla extract
1 teaspoon raw honey

1. Warm the nut milk in a small pot or a milk steamer.

2. Place the charcoal in a mug and slowly, while stirring, add the warm water and warm nut milk. Add the vanilla and honey.

3. Stir until well combined and sip.

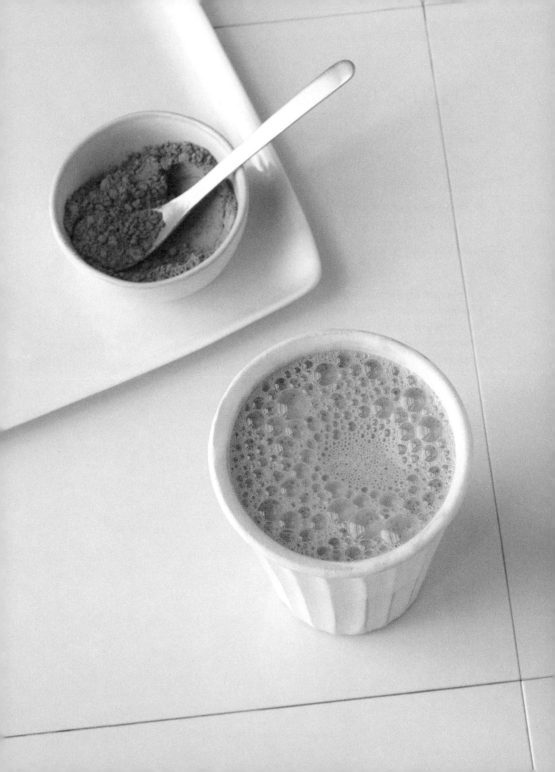

GOOD MOOD MATCHA

Antioxidant Boost, Mood, Skin

This cup of matcha may indeed lift your mood and give you an energy boost, all while tasting totally luscious and delicious. This is my personal go-to, everyday recipe. No fuss, totally yummy—and it delivers!

Makes 1 serving

1 teaspoon matcha powder
1 heaping tablespoon coconut butter
10 ounces warm (not boiling) water
¼ teaspoon ground cinnamon
1 teaspoon *Mucuna pruriens*
1 teaspoon reishi
1 scoop marine collagen peptides
1 teaspoon raw honey

1. Place all the ingredients in a blender that tolerates warm liquids. I like to use a mesh strainer for the matcha and add it slowly to avoid any lumps, but if you're in a rush, just throw everything in, close the lid, and blend it all up.

2. Pour into a beautiful mug and sip slowly.

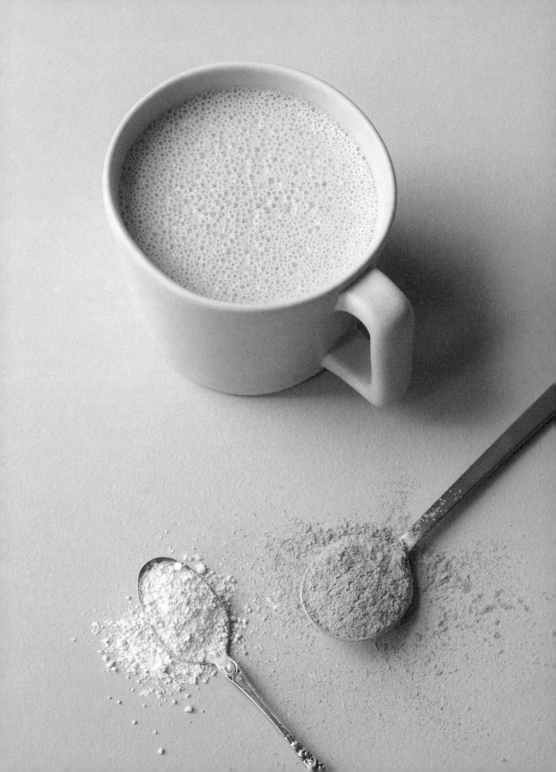

TAHINI MACA LATTE

Harmony, Hormone Balance, Beauty Boost

The creamy richness in this recipe comes from tahini, a sesame seed paste that is loaded with calcium and healthy fats. This creamy, sweet, and luscious drink is a real treat, and with maca and pearl, you'll feel glowing and harmonized to boot.

Makes 1 serving

1 tablespoon tahini
2 Medjool dates, pitted
1/4 teaspoon ground cinnamon,
   plus more for garnish
1/8 teaspoon sea salt
1/4 teaspoon maca
1/4 teaspoon pearl powder
1 cup warm water

1. Place all the ingredients, except the warm water, in a blender that tolerates warm liquids, then pour the water on top. Blend on high speed until frothy and creamy.

2. Pour into a cup, sprinkle with cinnamon, and enjoy!

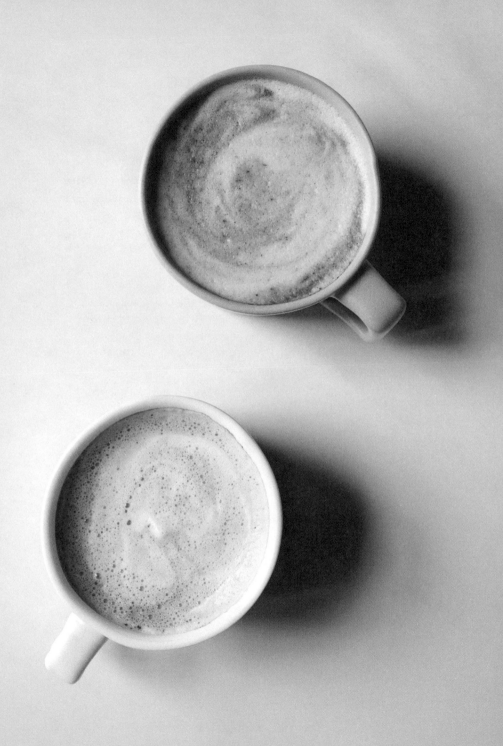

PINK LATTE

Blood Sugar Balance, Digestive Support, Heart Health

This is not just a pretty drink! That beautiful pink hue hints at some amazing antioxidant powers and heart support hiding within. The powdered beets are great for blood purification and stamina. Ginger and cinnamon provide digestive and blood sugar support, and both the hawthorn berries and beets are known to support the heart.

Makes 1 serving

1 teaspoon beet powder
1 teaspoon hawthorn berry
  powder
½ teaspoon ground ginger
½ teaspoon ground cinnamon
1 teaspoon raw honey
½ cup warm water
¾ cup nut milk (page 100),
  warmed

1. Place all the powders and honey in a mug or bowl and mix.

2. Add the warm water and whisk or blend with a hand-held milk frother until the powders have dissolved. Top with the warm nut milk.

BLUE LATTE

Beauty, Energy, Libido

The color of this drink seems truly unreal and magical. The blue comes from a blue algae rich in chlorophyll. The cashew milk makes the drink dreamy creamy and the hit of adaptogens provide rejuvenation and brain food.

Makes 1 serving

1 cup cashew milk (page 100)
1/2 teaspoon Blue Majik
1/2 teaspoon vanilla extract
1/2 teaspoon pine pollen
1/2 teaspoon amla
1 teaspoon raw honey

1. Place the milk in a small pot and gently warm (be careful not to bring to a boil). A milk warmer or frother will do the trick, too!

2. Place the powders in a mug and, while whisking, slowly pour in the warmed milk.

3. Add the honey and stir. Sip and feel the joy.

BEAUTY MOON MILK

Sleep, Beauty, Calming

A warming cup of creamy and sweet moon milk is just what you need before bed to help your body relax, release, and calm down from a busy day. This beverage is loaded with adaptogens that are sleep inducing, serotonin boosting, and helpful for unwinding from stressful days.

Makes 1 serving

1 tablespoon coconut butter
⅛ teaspoon ground cardamom
1 Medjool date, pitted
10 ounces warm water
Pinch of shatawari
Pinch of ashwagandha
Pinch of He Shou Wu
Pinch of *Mucuna pruriens*

1. Place all the ingredients in a blender.

2. Blend on high speed until the date is dissolved and the drink is well mixed.

3. Pour, sip, and enjoy.

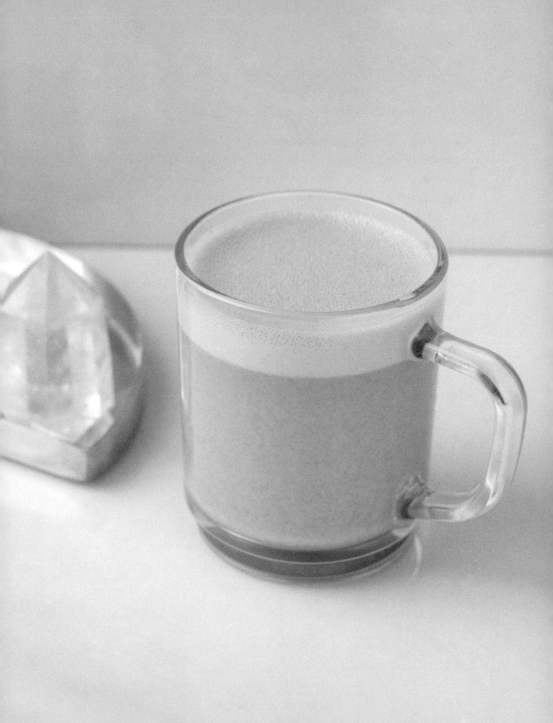

GOLDEN LATTE

Anti-Inflammatory, Digestive Support, Healing

When you want a warming, comforting drink in the morning, but caffeine is not agreeing with you—this is what you want. The spices give this a great, comforting flavor and they carry amazing anti-inflammatory benefits.

Makes 1 serving

1 tablespoon almond butter or sunflower butter
1 scoop collagen peptides
1 teaspoon raw manuka honey
2 teaspoons coconut oil
1/2 teaspoon astragalus
1/2 teaspoon reishi
1/8 teaspoon ground nutmeg
1/8 teaspoon ground cardamom
1/8 teaspoon ground cloves
1/8 teaspoon ground cinnamon
1/2 teaspoon ground turmeric
Pinch of pink Himalayan sea salt
1/8 teaspoon freshly ground black pepper
1/2 cup warm water
1/2 cup unsweetened almond milk (page 100), warmed

1. Combine all the ingredients in a blender and blend on high speed until creamy and frothy.

2. Pour into a mug and drink.

Pro Tip: For an iced version, blend all the ingredients together, using cold milk and water, and pour over ice.

REISHI HOT CHOCOLATE

Comfort and Calm, Immunity Support

Trust me, this is what your body wants on a cold afternoon. The high antioxidant content of chocolate helps protect your body from wintery colds and the creamy milk contains protein and fat, which your body needs more of to stay warm throughout winter.

Makes 1 serving

1 cup coconut milk (page 98) or any other milk of choice
1 teaspoon coconut oil
1 tablespoon raw cacao powder
2 tablespoons pure maple syrup
1/4 teaspoon vanilla powder or vanilla extract
1/2 teaspoon reishi

1. Place the milk and coconut oil in a small pot and heat until warm.

2. Transfer the warm milk to a blender along with the rest of the ingredients.

3. Blend on low speed until all is combined.

4. Pour into a mug and enjoy.

MAYAN HOT CHOCOLATE

Pleasure Boost, Aphrodisiac, Energy

Using real melted dark chocolate makes this drink extra-decadent, thick, and luscious. It has a little surprise kick in it, too! Treat yourself with antioxidants all around, healthy fats, stress relief, a dopamine boost, and a great mood boost from chocolate and *Mucuna pruriens*!

Serves 1 (or split it with a friend for a slightly smaller indulgence)

3 ounces chopped dark chocolate (I use 70% cacao. You could use stone-ground Mexican chocolate if you want to be really authentic and fancy!)
1 cup nut milk (page 100)
⅛ teaspoon chili powder (cayenne pepper would also work here)
¼ teaspoon ground cinnamon
¼ teaspoon ashwagandha
¼ teaspoon maca
¼ teaspoon *Mucuna pruriens*
Optional: a few red pepper flakes or marshmallows to sprinkle on top

1. Place the chocolate in a small pot and melt over low heat.

2. Warm the nut milk in a separate small pot and stir the warmed milk into the melted chocolate.

3. Whisk in all the powders.

4. Pour into small mugs, top with your garnish of choice, if using, and sip very slowly with your eyes closed.

COLDBREW ICED LATTE

Mood, Focus, Beauty

I love the smoothness of a cold-brewed iced coffee and, even better, the cold brew process makes for a much less acidic drink, too! This one is decked out with mood-boosting and stress-lowering adaptogens as well as the beloved pearl powder for glowing skin.

Makes 1 serving

½ cup cold-brewed coffee
½ cup almond milk (page 100)
¼ teaspoon pearl powder
¼ teaspoon *Mucuna pruriens*
Pinch of ashwagandha

1. Place all the ingredients in a glass and use a small hand-held electric whisk to mix everything together.

2. Add ice and a glass straw. Sip in the sun!

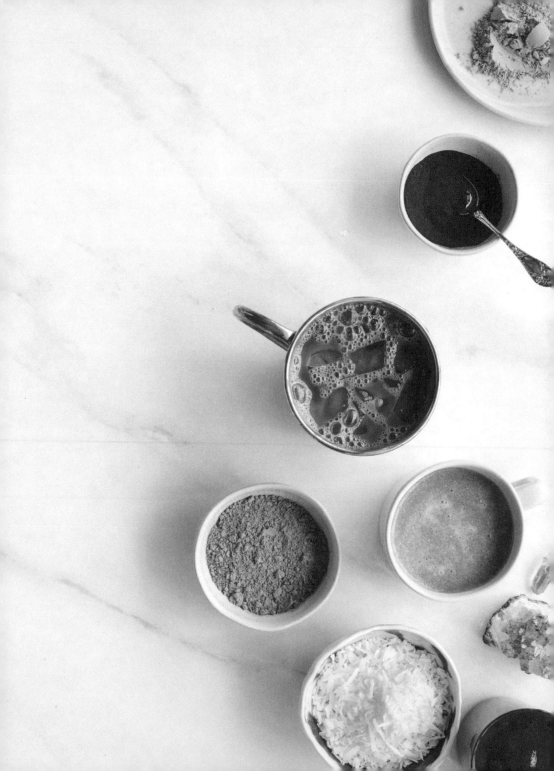

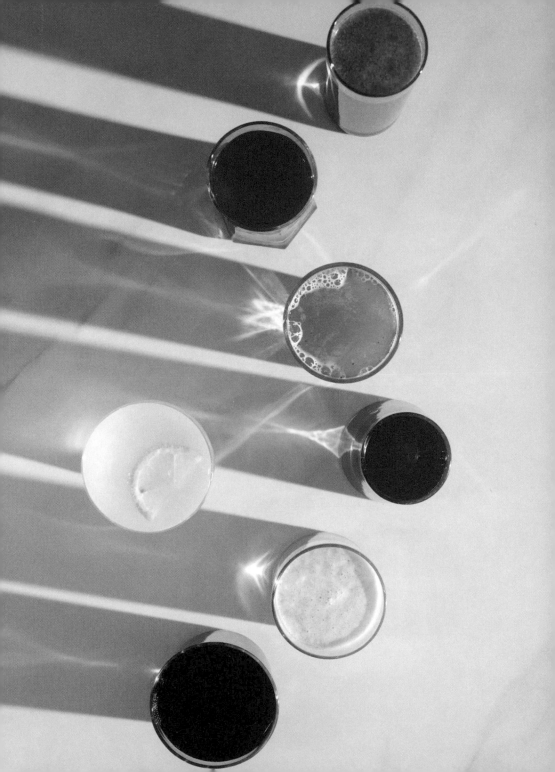

TONICS

Tonic drinks are traditionally toning drinks for health and wellness. *Toning* is a word used in Chinese medicine to describe herbs that are supporting and can help build up and strengthen in a preventative way. These herbal concoctions for healing, health, and well-being are worth incorporating into your self-care routine. They also make for great nonalcoholic drink alternatives when you want something more than water but without the downside of headaches and sluggishness the next day.

121

ADRENAL TONIC

Harmony, Hydration, Adrenal Support

Real salt is very important for your adrenal glands, and a common symptom of what's often called adrenal fatigue is . . . salt cravings! Actual sea salt (and especially pink Himalayan sea salt, Celtic sea salt, and the Real Salt brand) contains trace minerals that your body needs badly. Real mineral-rich salts also help with proper absorption of the water you're drinking. This drink is a great way to start the day.

Makes 1 serving

1 cup filtered water
Juice of ½ lemon
¼ teaspoon pink Himalayan sea
   salt
1 teaspoon baobab powder or
   another natural vitamin C
   powder
¼ teaspoon ashwagandha

Mix all the ingredients together in a glass and drink.

BEAUTY TONIC

Beauty, Love, Rejuvenating

Packed with beauty-boosting powders, this is sure to make you glow from within!

Makes 1 serving

½ cup unsweetened
  pomegranate juice
Juice of ½ lime
¼ teaspoon pearl powder
½ teaspoon rose water
¼ teaspoon amla
½ cup sparkling water

1. Mix the juices and powders together in a glass.

2. Top with the sparkling water.

ORANGES & CREAM

Energy, Anti-Inflammatory, Immunity

Sweet and slightly creamy with a throwback to childhood, this elixir is refreshing, energy boosting, and anti-inflammatory.

Makes 1 serving

3/4 cup fresh orange juice
2 tablespoons coconut cream
1/2 teaspoon reishi
1/2 teaspoon ground turmeric

This drink might benefit from a quick whirl in a blender to properly dissolve the coconut cream and powders, but in a pinch, a small handheld electric whisk will do the trick.

QUENCHER

Hydration, Energy, Digestive Support

This red elixir is energy and electrolyte packed. With red berries' antioxidant power, probiotics for skin and gut health, as well as hydrating coconut water, this is a great alternative to any old sports drink after a sweat session.

Makes 1 serving

¼ cup coconut water
1 tablespoon probiotic coconut water (inner-ēco brand or similar)
1 teaspoon goji powder
¼ teaspoon Schisandra berry powder
¼ teaspoon rhodiola
¾ cup sparkling water

1. Mix the coconut waters and powders together in a glass.

2. Top with the sparkling water.

BLUE LAGOON LEMONADE

Mood, Energy, Detox

This is an up-leveled lemonade with clean and nourishing ingredients. Raw honey is the only sweetener and the blue hue is of course from nature's own blue algae.

Makes 1 serving

1 teaspoon raw honey
A little warm water
Juice of 1 lemon
½ teaspoon Blue Majik
¼ teaspoon *Mucuna pruriens*
1 cup filtered water

1. Dissolve the honey in a glass with the warm water, add the lemon juice and powders, and mix well.

2. Top with the water and drink.

NIGHTCAP TONIC

Sleep, Calming, Stress Relief

Sip on this tonic before bedtime for an easy transition into sleep. Tart cherry juice is not only totally delicious, but it contains natural melatonin—the hormone for sleep and circadian rhythm regulation.

Makes 1 serving

½ cup tart cherry juice
½ teaspoon ashwagandha
¼ cup filtered or sparkling water

1. Stir the juice and powder together in a glass.

2. Top with the water and enjoy.

HEART TONIC

Heart Health, Calming, Anti-Inflammatory

This tonic contains only good things for your heart and blood. Hibiscus can help lower blood pressure, beet is a blood cleanser, and cinnamon helps with blood sugar regulation. Hawthorn is an ancient heart-supporting adaptogen and rose water is believed to balance the heart.

Makes 1 serving

1 cup steeped hibiscus tea, allowed to cool
1/2 teaspoon rose water
1/4 teaspoon hawthorn berry powder
1/2 teaspoon beet powder
1/4 teaspoon ground cinnamon
1/2 teaspoon pure maple syrup

1. Combine all the ingredients in a glass, stirring well to make sure the syrup and powders mix and dissolve.

2. Add ice if you want to, and enjoy!

DETOX TONIC

Cleansing, Detox Support, Clarity

This tonic is a variation on the classic lemon water cleanse: hydrating, spicy, sweet, and sour. Containing lemon, charcoal, and cayenne, this tonic is loaded with all the detox support your body desires, while the added adaptogens will provide some strength and stamina to help you make it through the day.

Makes 1 serving

½ teaspoon activated charcoal
Juice of 1 lemon
1 teaspoon pure maple syrup
Pinch of cayenne pepper
¼ teaspoon astragalus
¼ teaspoon rhodiola

1. Combine all the ingredients in a glass, stirring well to make sure the syrup and powders mix and dissolve.

2. Sip on an empty stomach.

WARM WINTER TISANE

Strength, Calmness, Stress Response

Winter requires warmth, self-care, and comfort! It's a time for looking inward, hibernating, and recharging. This warm tisane is nurturing and supports your body's immune system so that you can make it through the season with ease.

Makes 1 serving

1 holy basil tea bag, or 1 teaspoon loose leaves
1 cup hot water
1 tablespoon coconut cream or coconut milk (page 98)
1 teaspoon raw honey
¼ teaspoon ashwagandha
¼ teaspoon rhodiola
¼ teaspoon eleuthero

1. Steep the holy basil in the water, covered, for 10 minutes. Remove the tea bag or strain the tea.

2. Stir in the coconut cream, honey, and adaptogen powders.

3. Sip and enjoy.

TREATS

Welcome to everyone's favorite chapter—the treats with benefits! They are guilt-free pleasures (because guilt is such a waste of time and an all-around energy zapper I don't support!). Loaded with nutrient-dense, whole, real foods, these are desserts, bites, balls, and bars that you can feel good about eating any and every day. When our body is calm, comfortable, well rested, and nourished, we don't crave as much sugar and quick carbs. A well-nourished body has the nutrients and energy it needs to do all of its jobs! These treats are the means to that end, packed with delicious spices, chocolate, natural sweetness, and, of course, nutrient-dense super powders! And don't miss the seriously awesome popcorn recipe.

UNBEATABLE BROWNIES

Antioxidant Boost, Calming, Mood

Slightly bitter, like really dark chocolate. Loaded with fiber, healthy fats, antioxidants, and adaptogenic power. Yeah, these brownies might make you feel unbeatable and unstoppable.

Makes 8 brownies

1 cup Medjool dates, pitted
1 cup raw walnuts
2 tablespoons raw cacao powder, plus more for dusting
1/2 teaspoon pink Himalayan sea salt
1/4 teaspoon ground cinnamon
1/2 teaspoon vanilla extract
1 teaspoon ashwagandha
1 tablespoon maca
1/4 cup chocolate chips (or chop up your favorite chocolate bar!)
Optional: chocolate sauce

1. Place all the ingredients, except the chocolate chips and sauce, in a food processor and process until well combined into a crumbly "dough."

2. Pour into an 8-inch square glass container and add the chocolate chips.

3. Press the mixture into an even, 1-inch-thick layer in the container. Let cool in the fridge for 30 minutes to 1 hour.

4. Dust the brownies with cacao powder and cut into 2-inch squares.

5. Drizzle with chocolate sauce, if you want!

CHOCOLATE BARK WITH GOJI BERRIES AND ROSE PETALS

Energy, Brain Boost, Focus

Yeah—you can absolutely make your own chocolate! This beautiful bark contains rose petals and energizing goji berries. Make it as your own self-care treat, or gift it to someone special in your life.

Makes 8 pieces/servings

¼ cup coconut oil, at room temperature
¼ cup ghee, at room temperature
1 cup raw cacao powder
½ teaspoon pink Himalayan sea salt
¼ cup raw honey or pure maple syrup
2 teaspoons pine pollen
1 teaspoon rhodiola
2 tablespoons goji berries
Culinary-grade rose petals, crushed (optional)
1 tablespoon cacao nibs

1. Make sure the coconut oil and ghee are soft or liquid, then mix them well in a medium bowl. If needed, you can gently melt the coconut oil over low heat or hot water.

2. Add the cacao powder, salt, and honey and stir well before adding the pine pollen and rhodiola.

3. Pour the chocolate mixture into an 8-inch square glass dish, or you can shape aluminum foil into a rectangular shape with a 2-inch rim and use that! This is supposed to look like a homemade treat so just improvise and use what you have on hand.

continued

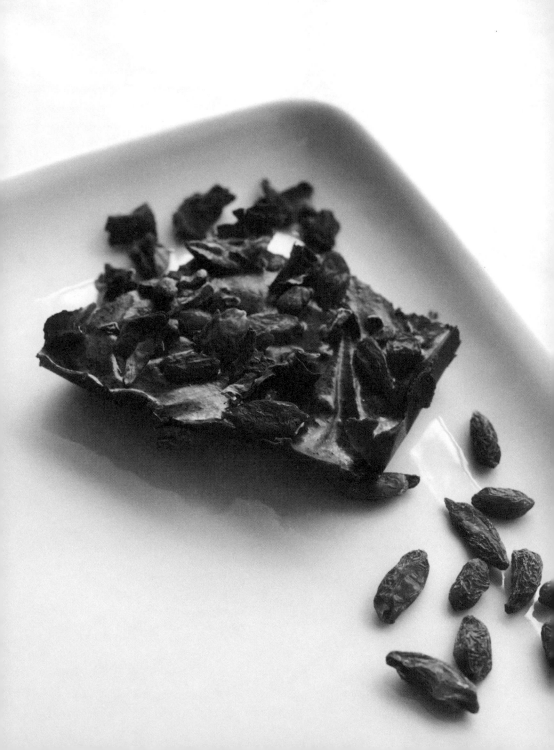

4. Sprinkle crushed rose petals, if using, and the cacao nibs over the chocolate mixture.

5. Let set in the freezer for 30 minutes or more.

6. Remove the bark from the mold and, using your hands, break it into rough pieces.

7. Eat right away or store in the fridge.

135

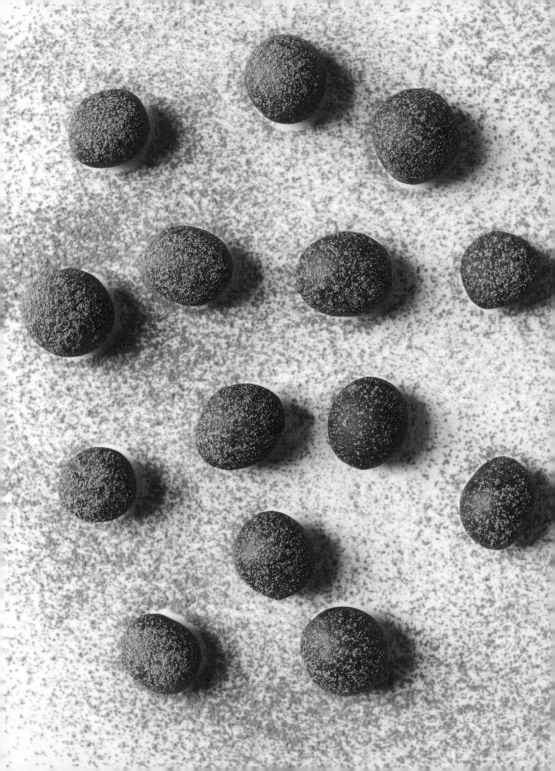

WOMEN'S BONBONS

Women's Health, Skin, Metabolism

These little bites are packed with flavor and just a few will provide you with a nice boost of energy and well-being. They offer collagen, pearl, and coconut butter for the skin; cinnamon and cayenne for a metabolism boost; and adaptogens to help balance hormones and keep your cool.

Makes 10 bonbons

10 ounces dark chocolate
2 tablespoons coconut cream
1 vanilla bean
2 scoops collagen peptides
1/2 teaspoon astragalus
1/2 teaspoon He Shou Wu
1/2 teaspoon pearl powder
1/2 teaspoon ground cinnamon
1/8 teaspoon cayenne pepper
1/4 teaspoon sea salt
1/2 cup raw cacao powder for rolling and dusting

1. Place the chocolate and coconut cream in a small pot and melt over low heat.

2. Split the vanilla bean lengthwise down the front and scrape out the seeds using the back of a knife. Add the seeds to the melted chocolate mixture.

3. Stir in the remaining ingredients and refrigerate for 1 to 2 hours, until set but still malleable. The mix will feel firm but sticky and still easy to roll into balls.

4. Coat your hands with cacao powder and roll the mixture into 10 1-inch balls, placing them on a parchment-lined baking sheet or plate.

5. Refrigerate for 10 to 15 minutes, then dust with more cacao powder!

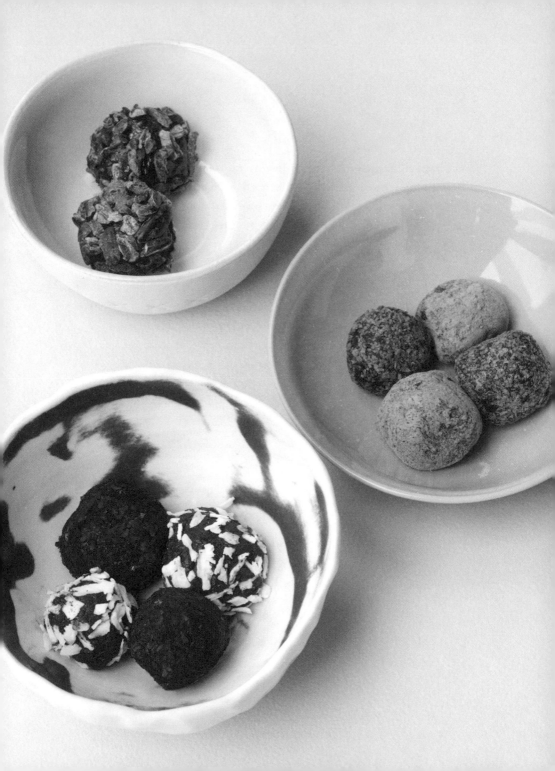

YOUR TRUFFLES

Energy, Hormone Balance, Stress Relief

We all have individual needs and tastes, so I created these truffles to be completely customizable! Make the base, add your adaptogens or powders of choice, and roll the truffles in any topping your heart desires.

Makes 12 balls

¼ cup coconut oil
½ cup raw cacao powder
¼ cup honey or pure maple syrup
2 pinches of sea salt
1 tablespoon nut milk (page 100), chilled
¼ to ½ teaspoon of each adaptogen of choice
Your choice of toppings (my favorites include cacao nibs, freeze-dried raspberry powder, cacao powder, shredded coconut, hemp seeds, or sesame seeds!)

1. Warm the coconut oil in a small container (should hold at least 1 cup) in a hot water bath.

2. Remove the oil from the bath and add the cacao powder, honey, salt, and your adaptogen powders of choice. Stir until well combined.

3. Add the cold nut milk and mix. Add more cacao or milk, as desired.

4. Let sit in the fridge for 10 minutes to allow the mixture to harden slightly. Check periodically to make sure it doesn't get too solid.

5. Roll the sticky mixture into 12 balls and roll the balls in your topping of choice.

6. Place on a tray in the fridge to set (10 to 15 minutes), or place in the freezer for an even faster path to eating!

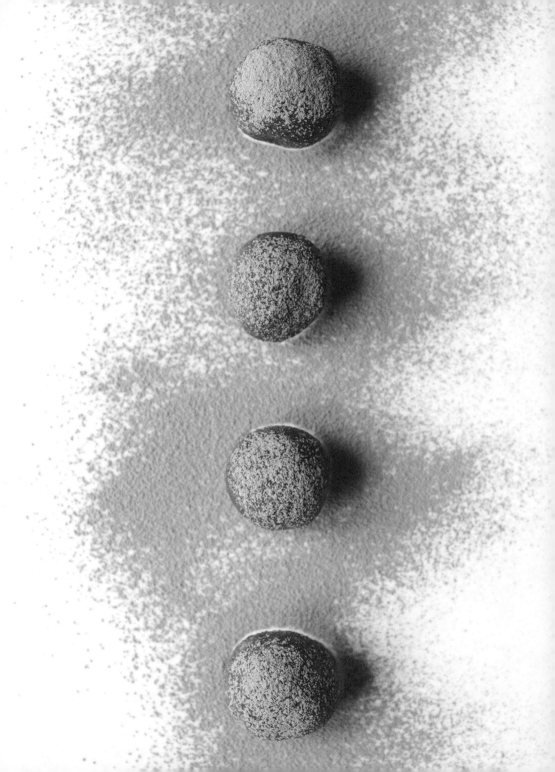

MATCHA BLISS BALLS

Skin, Hormone Balance, Immunity Boost

Fully loaded with healthy fats and antioxidants, just one of these balls will provide you with an energy boost and some stress and immunity support. They are not too sweet and make a great snack that will tide you over before your next meal. I love storing these in the freezer, for freshness, coolness, and texture.

Makes 10 to 12 balls

¼ cup pumpkin seeds
¼ cup pistachios
½ cup cashews
½ cup almonds
1 cup unsweetened shredded coconut
1 teaspoon ground cinnamon
¼ teaspoon sea salt
2 tablespoons matcha powder, plus more for dusting (optional)
½ cup coconut oil
¼ cup coconut butter
⅓ cup almond milk (page 100) or coconut milk (page 98)
4 Medjool dates, pitted
2 teaspoons astragalus
2 teaspoons reishi
2 tablespoons manuka honey

1. Place all the ingredients in a food processor.

2. Pulse until well combined. It should be a pulverized, sticky mixture.

3. With clean hands, roll the mixture into 2-inch balls.

4. Place the balls on a baking sheet or plate and place in the freezer.

5. Store in an airtight container in the fridge or freezer.

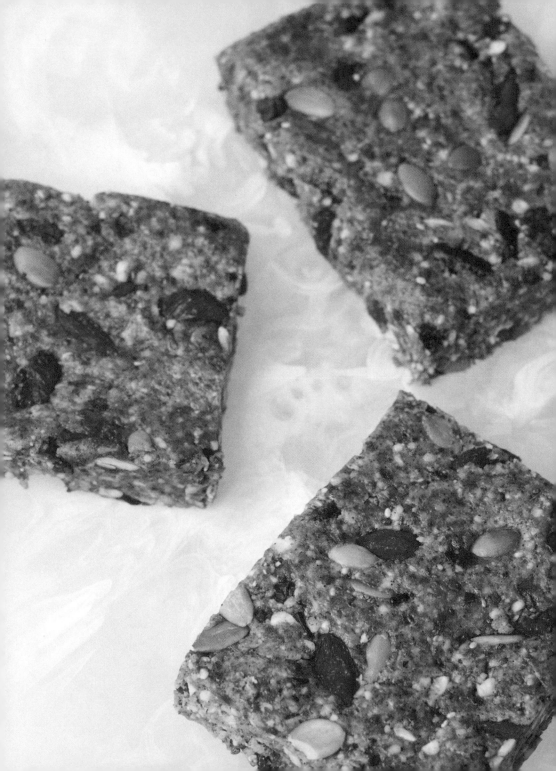

ENERGY BARS

Sustenance, Hormone Balance, Energy

There are lots of so-called energy bars, protein bars, and granola bars on the market, and one thing most of them have in common is way too much sugar and too many ingredients. This energy bar is unlike any other energy bar. It provides long-lasting energy and lots of nutrients to fuel your body well. It's got protein, good fats, fiber, and carbohydrates, so it's a perfect on-the-go snack or small meal. Dates are a great energy food loaded with fiber, potassium, and natural sweetness, and goji berries are a celebrated energizing superfood! Maca adds a nice butterscotch flavor and a boost of hormone balance and energy.

Makes 6 bars

1 cup Medjool dates, pitted
1/4 cup cashews
1/4 cup hazelnuts
1/4 cup almonds
1/4 cup almond butter
1 tablespoon coconut oil
1/2 teaspoon pink Himalayan sea salt
Seeds of 1 vanilla bean
1 tablespoon goji powder
1 1/2 teaspoons maca
2 tablespoons collagen peptides
1 tablespoon chia seeds
3 tablespoons goji berries
3 tablespoons pumpkin seeds
3 tablespoons cacao nibs

1. Line a baking dish or board with parchment paper.

2. Place the dates, nuts, almond butter, oil, and salt in a food processor and pulse until chopped and well combined.

3. Add the vanilla seeds, goji and maca powders, collagen, and chia seeds and pulse until well combined.

4. Pour into a medium bowl and mix in the goji berries, pumpkin seeds, and cacao nibs. It's easiest to just use your hands to mix here.

continued

5. Pour the mixture into the prepared baking dish, spreading it into a 1-inch-thick rectangle.

6. Place in the freezer for 20 minutes, or in the fridge for 1 to 2 hours to let set, then cut into six rectangular bars or, if you prefer, smaller cubes.

7. Wrap each bar individually with parchment paper and store in the fridge, so you can grab one when you're on the go or need a pick-me-up!

CHOCOLATE MILKSHAKE

Stress Relief, Beauty, Energy

Who doesn't love a thick, creamy, and cool chocolate shake? And this one is certainly good for you, too! It's jam-packed with good fats, fiber, minerals, and antioxidants as well as stress-busting adaptogens!

Makes 1 serving

1 1/4 cups cashew milk (page 100)
1 tablespoon raw cacao powder
1 tablespoon chia seeds
1/2 frozen banana
1/2 frozen avocado
1 Medjool date, pitted
1/4 teaspoon He Shou Wu
1/4 teaspoon ashwagandha
1/4 teaspoon Schisandra berry powder

1. Place all the ingredients in a high-powered blender.

2. Blend until well combined, thick, and luscious.

3. Pour into a tall glass and sip, or eat with a spoon.

Pro Tip: Whenever your bananas and avocados are close to being overly ripe, peel them, cut them in halves or quarters, and freeze for easy use later in smoothies, bowls, and shakes!

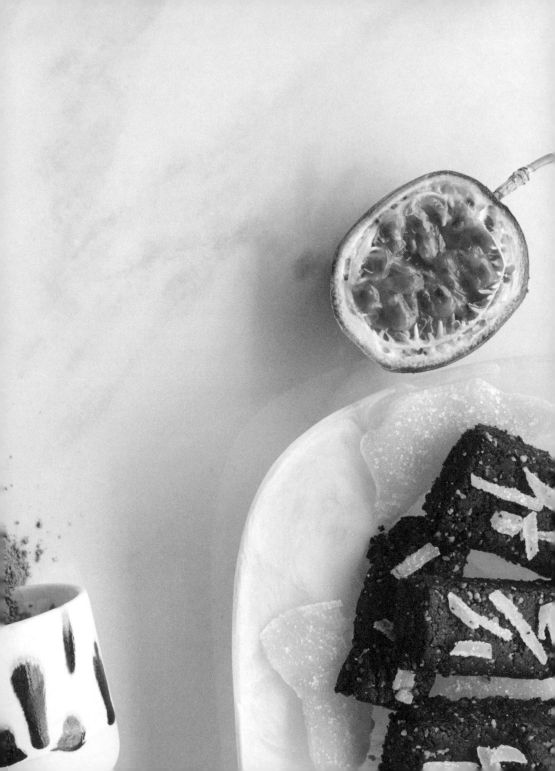

NO-COOK CHOCOLATE GINGER SQUARES

Elevated Mood, Well-being, Immunity Boost

This delicious treat includes only the best parts of gingerbread cookies—the chewiness, the spices, and that little kick of ginger! All without the wheat flour or white sugar. These are spiked with *Mucuna pruriens* for a massive mood boost, and ashwagandha for all-around awesomeness and resilience!

Makes 8 squares

DRY MIXTURE
1 cup walnuts
1/2 cup almond flour
1/4 cup coconut flour
1/2 cup raw cacao powder
1 teaspoon ground ginger
1 teaspoon ground cinnamon
1/4 teaspoon ground cardamom
1/4 teaspoon ground cloves
1/4 teaspoon sea salt
1/8 teaspoon freshly ground
    black pepper
1 teaspoon ashwagandha
1 teaspoon *Mucuna pruriens*
1/4 cup candied ginger, plus more
    to decorate on top

WET MIXTURE
1 cup Medjool dates, pitted
1 tablespoon ghee
1 teaspoon vanilla extract
2 tablespoons molasses

1. Prepare the dry mixture: Stir together all the dry ingredients in a medium bowl.

2. Transfer the dry mixture to a food processor and add the dates, ghee, vanilla, and molasses. Pulse until well mixed. The mixture will look crumbly and a bit dry.

3. Line an 8-inch square baking dish or pan with parchment paper and press the mixture into it, using your fists. The mixture will stick together. Place in the fridge for an hour to set.

4. Once the mixture has set, decorate with thin strips or small chunks of candied ginger. Cut into squares. Store in the fridge.

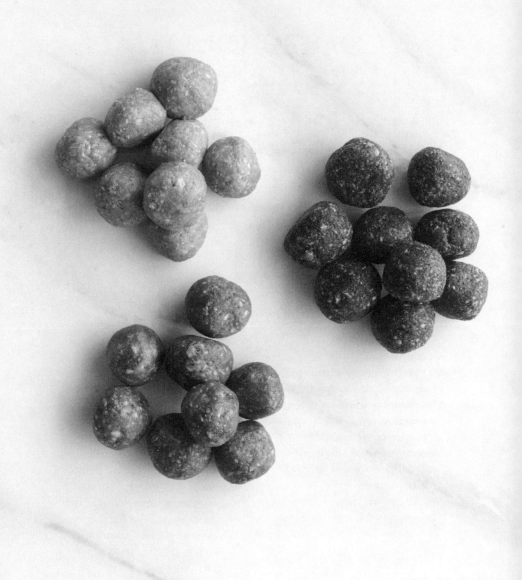

RAW MACAROONS FOUR WAYS

Hormone Balance, Energy, Adrenal Health

Macaroons make for tasty treats that look really cute, too. All the coconut in these provides healthy fats, which is good for your hormone balance, skin, and energy levels. Once you've made the base, you can choose which variations you want to make based on your preference or what you happen to have on hand.

Makes 10 macaroons

BASE
- 1 cup unsweetened shredded coconut
- 1/2 cup almond flour
- 1/4 teaspoon pink Himalayan sea salt
- 2 tablespoons pure maple syrup or coconut nectar
- 2 tablespoons coconut oil
- 1 teaspoon vanilla extract

VARIATIONS

GREEN
- 2 tablespoons moringa leaf powder
- 1 teaspoon matcha powder

GOLDEN
- 2 tablespoons ground turmeric
- 1/2 teaspoon ground cinnamon
- 1/4 teaspoon ground cardamom

PINK
- 1 tablespoon goji powder
- 1 tablespoon beet powder
- 2 teaspoons pine pollen

BROWN
- 2 tablespoons raw cacao powder
- 1 tablespoon maca
- 1 tablespoon cacao nibs
- Melted chocolate for dipping (optional)

MINT CHIP
- 2 tablespoons cacao nibs
- 4 drops peppermint extract
- 1 teaspoon astragalus

continued

1. To make the base, place the dry ingredients in a bowl and stir in the coconut oil, maple syrup, and vanilla. (If the coconut oil is hard at room temperature, gently melt it over low heat or in a hot water bath.)

2. Stir until all the ingredients are well combined.

3. Add your chosen flavor variation and mix well.

4. Roll the mixture into 2-inch balls.

5. Place the balls on a baking sheet or tray and place in the freezer for 20 minutes or more.

6. Transfer the firm balls to an airtight container and store in the fridge or freezer for a couple of weeks.

SPOONFULS

Energy, Digestion, Mood Boost

This is the perfect spoonful when you need a little boost! Maybe it's that moment when you walk in the door at home after a long day at work and you need a little something before tackling dinner, kids, or a workout. Or maybe it's the first thing you grab in the morning—either way, this rich, luscious, ganache-like supermixture will hit the spot with a hint of heat, lots of adaptogens, and anti-inflammatory benefits.

Makes about 8 ounces (1 cup)

½ cup coconut butter
¼ cup ghee
1 tablespoon manuka honey
¼ cup raw cacao powder
½ teaspoon ground cinnamon
½ teaspoon ground ginger
½ teaspoon ground turmeric
¼ teaspoon ground cardamom
⅛ teaspoon pink Himalayan sea salt
1 teaspoon ashwagandha
½ teaspoon astragalus
½ teaspoon He Shou Wu
1 teaspoon *Mucuna pruriens*

1. Stir together the coconut butter, ghee, and honey in a bowl until well combined.

2. Add the powders while stirring gently to combine the mixture well.

3. Store in an airtight jar.

4. Eat 1 teaspoon at a time—either on its own or spread on toast, crackers, or fruit.

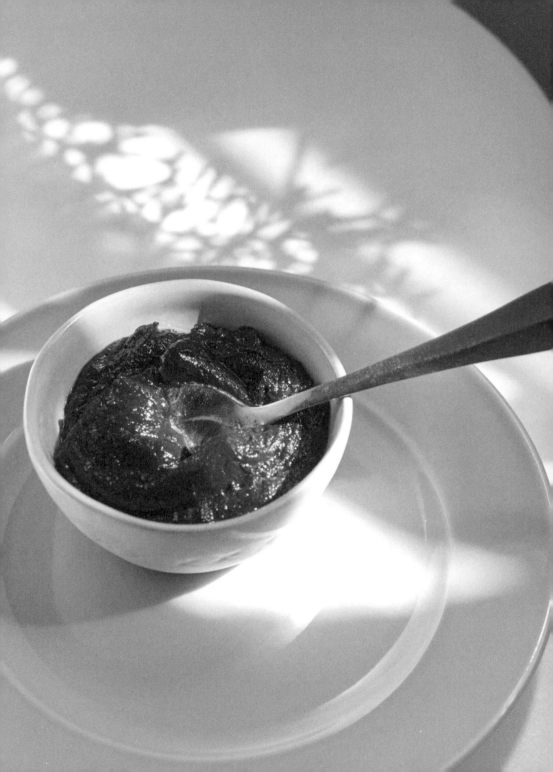

TAHINI SHROOMS CHOCOLATE SPREAD

Immunity, Brain Boost, Antioxidant Power

This spread is great on toast; drizzled over a bowl of fresh berries, oatmeal, or ice cream; or, of course, straight out of the jar. It may remind you of a certain European chocolate spread, but this version is free of nasty oils and processed sugar and loaded with good fats, calcium, minerals, and antioxidants.

Makes about 12 ounces (1 1/2 cups)

1 cup tahini
1/3 cup raw cacao powder
1/3 cup pure maple syrup
1/4 teaspoon pink Himalayan sea salt
1 teaspoon vanilla extract
1/2 teaspoon chaga
1/2 teaspoon lion's mane
1/2 teaspoon reishi
1/2 teaspoon cordyceps

1. Stir together all the ingredients in a medium bowl until well combined.

2. Store in a 12-ounce glass jar in the fridge. It could last for weeks in the fridge, but you will probably finish it way before then.

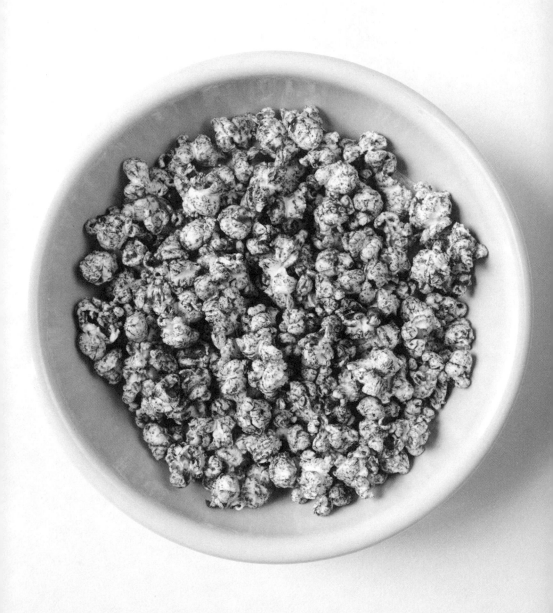

GREEN POPCORN

Calming, Immunity, Supports Healing

Sometimes nothing quite hits the spot or provides more "chillaxing" comfort than a bowl of salty, crunchy popcorn. And when you make it yourself, with good fats and some super powders, it can be a worthwhile treat. Enjoy with your favorite movie for the ultimate wellness experience.

Makes 2 servings (but I won't judge if you eat it all by yourself!)

1 tablespoon ghee for popping
¼ cup organic popcorn kernels
¼ cup olive oil or ghee for coating
¼ teaspoon pink Himalayan sea salt
2 teaspoons garlic powder
Pinch of cayenne powder
1 teaspoon chlorella or spirulina
½ teaspoon reishi

1. Place the tablespoon of ghee in a large, lidded pot over medium heat and let it melt.

2. Add a few corn kernels and close the lid. Once they pop, add the rest of the popcorn.

3. Keep shaking and moving the pot a bit while the corn pops. Once the popping slows down, lower the heat while allowing any remaining kernels to pop.

4. While the corn is popping, heat the ¼ cup of oil in a small pot. Remove from the heat and add the salt, garlic powder, and cayenne. Let cool slightly before adding the chlorella and reishi.

5. Transfer the oil mixture to a serving bowl. Pour in the popcorn and toss until it is coated and has a nice green color.

6. Eat up!

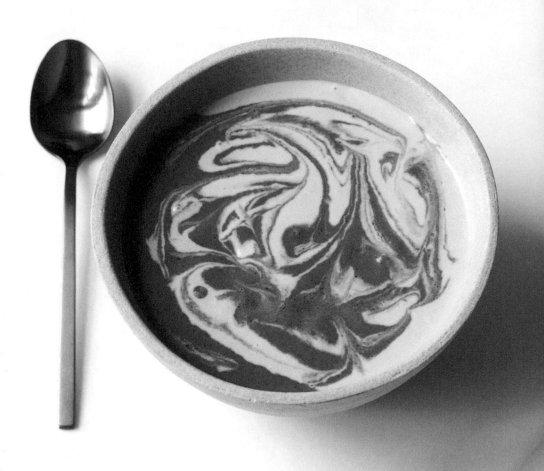

GOOD MORNING RECIPES

Bowls, smoothies, and pumped-up granola are here to help you start your day with vibrant, nourishing, and powered-up foods. Then, go through your day like a superhuman!

The smoothies in this section have everything your body needs to start the day off right: protein, fiber, healthy fats, and energy-boosting super powders! Breaking the fast with the right foods gets you off to great start and gives you stable fuel and uplifting energy for the day ahead.

UNICORN BOWL

Beauty, Immunity, Antioxidant Power

This bowl is not just bright and beautiful eye candy, it's also full of good-for-you plants and fats that will power you up for the day. The pink color comes from dragon fruit—the fruit of the pitaya cactus plant—which is a true superfood full of antioxidants, good fats, minerals, vitamins, and fiber. The blue is from the amazing algae Blue Majik, a plant source of complete protein packed with antioxidants and energizing B vitamins.

Serves 2

BLEND 1
One 2-ounce package frozen
   coconut meat
1/2 frozen banana
One 100-gram package frozen
   dragon fruit
1/4 cup frozen mango
1/2 cup coconut water
1/4 teaspoon hawthorn berry
   powder
1/4 teaspoon Schisandra berry
   powder

BLEND 2
One 2-ounce package frozen
   coconut meat
1 frozen banana
1/2 cup coconut milk (page 98) or
   any plant milk of your choice
1/2 teaspoon vanilla powder
1/2 teaspoon Blue Majik
1/4 teaspoon pearl powder
1/4 teaspoon reishi

Optional: Top with any of your
   favorite nuts, seeds, shredded
   coconut, granola, and fruit.

1. Make blend 1 by placing those ingredients in a blender and blending on high speed until smooth and well combined. Because all the ingredients are frozen, you might have to stop the blender and stir a few times and really work the mixture until it's blended. This is what gets you a thick smoothie bowl!

2. Pour blend 1 into a glass or small mug and set aside.

3. Rinse the blender.

4. Make blend 2 by placing those ingredients in the clean blender and blending on high speed until smooth and well combined. Again, do what it takes to make this thick mixture blend well.

5. Pour half of each blend simultaneously into a bowl—pouring blend 1 and blend 2 from opposite sides, at similar speed, so that half of the bowl is pink and the other half is blue. Repeat for the second bowl.

6. Using a chopstick or a spoon, carefully swirl and blend the two colors together to create a pretty pattern.

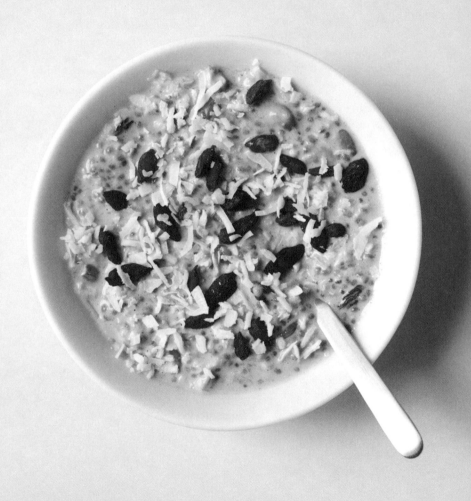

OVERNIGHT CHIA OATS

Digestion, Skin, Stable Energy

There is nothing that makes me feel more on top of things than when breakfast is prepared the night before and just waiting for me in the fridge! Overnight oats are so quick to toss together and make a truly filling, nourishing, and scrumptious breakfast—whether eaten at home or on the go!

Makes 1 large or 2 smaller servings

1 cup nut milk (page 100)
1/2 cup rolled oats
2 tablespoons chia seeds
2 tablespoons pumpkin seeds
1 ripe banana, mashed
1 teaspoon pure maple syrup
1/4 teaspoon ground cinnamon
1/4 teaspoon pink Himalayan sea salt
1 tablespoon goji berries, plus more for topping
1 tablespoon sea buckthorn powder

1. Mix all the ingredients together in either a bowl, jar, or container with a lid.

2. Place in the fridge overnight or for a few hours.

3. When ready to eat, top with some fresh berries, goji berries, and/or nuts of your choice.

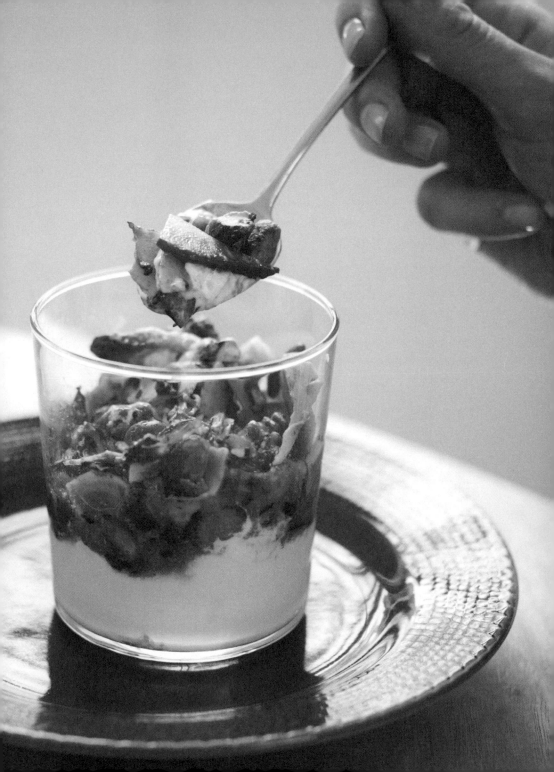

ADAPTOGENIC NUT-GRANOLA

Stamina, Stable Energy, Skin Glow

Granola is the original "health food" but often not very healthy, due to all the added sugars and oils. This recipe uses real food ingredients and delicious nuts and seeds full of minerals and healthy fats. Collagen peptides provide protein and the ashwagandha is there to help you tackle the day, no matter what life brings you. Use as a topping for yogurt or smoothies, or eat with some nut milk or simply as a snack.

Makes 3 cups (12 servings)

1 cup pistachios, roughly chopped
1 cup pecans, roughly chopped
3 tablespoons sesame seeds
1 cup coconut flakes
1 teaspoon pink Himalayan sea salt
1/2 teaspoon ground cinnamon
2 tablespoons collagen peptides
1 teaspoon ashwagandha
2 tablespoons coconut oil
1/4 cup pure maple syrup

1. Preheat the oven to 300°F.

2. Toss all the nuts, seeds, and coconut together in a bowl.

3. Add the salt, cinnamon, collagen, and ashwagandha and mix well.

4. Drizzle with the coconut oil and maple syrup and mix well.

5. Spread the granola mixture on a baking sheet and place in the oven.

6. Bake for 30 to 35 minutes, tossing the mixture every 10 minutes.

7. Remove the granola from the oven and let cool before transferring to an airtight jar.

MATCHA MILKSHAKE

Skin, Energy

This green smoothie is loaded with healthy fats, electrolytes, protein, greens, and alertness-boosting matcha! All you need, and more, for a complete breakfast in one truly delicious drink.

Makes 1 serving

1 cup coconut water
One 2-ounce package frozen
  coconut meat
1 cup spinach
½ avocado, peeled and pitted
1 date, for added sweetness
  (optional)
1 teaspoon matcha powder
1 tablespoon marine collagen
  peptides
½ teaspoon cordyceps
½ teaspoon reishi
Pinch of sea salt

Place all the ingredients in a blender and blend on high speed for about 1 minute, or until well combined.

GOLDEN SUNRISE SHAKE

Anti-Inflammatory, Digestion, Comfort Food

Smoothies are made for sunny mornings, and this blend is the perfect flavor combination for a crisp fall day. Warming spices help boost circulation and kick-start digestion. The beautiful orange hue is thanks to turmeric and pumpkin, which provide anti-inflammatory support, fiber, and comforting flavors.

Makes 1 serving

1 cup nut milk (page 100)
2 Medjool dates, pitted
1 tablespoon almond butter
1/2 cup pure pumpkin puree
1/4 teaspoon ground cinnamon
1/4 teaspoon astragalus
1/4 teaspoon ground turmeric
Freshly ground black pepper

Place all the ingredients in a blender, adding pepper to taste, and blend on high speed for about 1 minute, or until the dates have dissolved and the mixture is well combined.

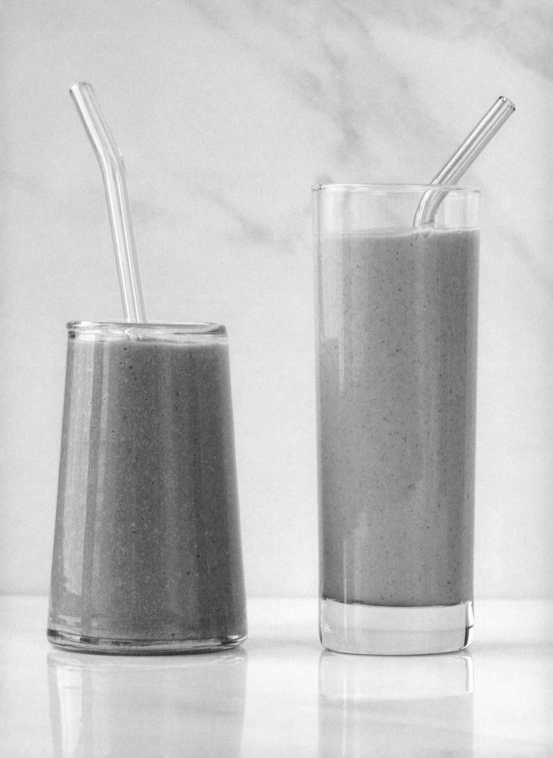

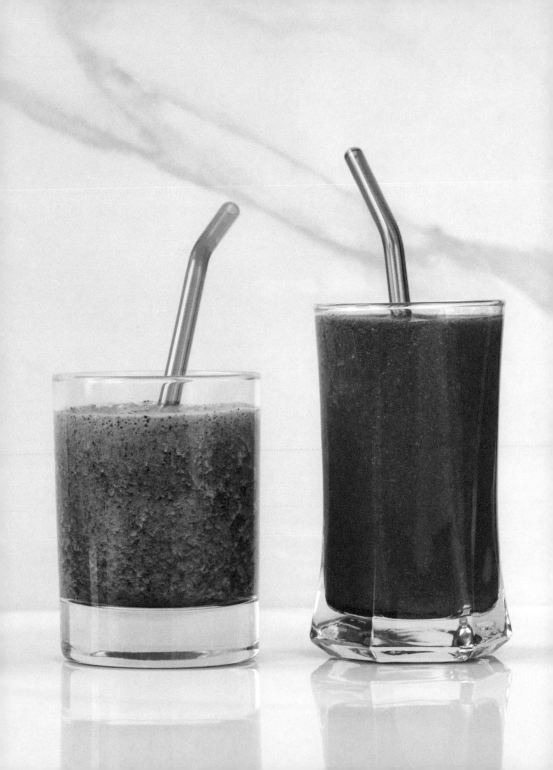

BLUE AGAINST BLUES

Energy, Beauty, Libido

The hue of this pretty smoothie is enough to inspire, and even on a cloudy day, it will remind you of blue skies and days at the beach. It's protein and antioxidant packed, with pearl for glowing skin and pine pollen for a libido boost!

Makes 1 serving

1 cup almond milk (page 100)
1/2 frozen banana
1/2 cup blueberries or frozen wild blueberries
1 tablespoon pea protein or collagen peptides
1/4 teaspoon astragalus
1/4 teaspoon pine pollen
1/4 teaspoon pearl powder
1/2 teaspoon Blue Majik
Pinch of sea salt

Place all the ingredients in a blender and blend on high speed for about 1 minute, or until well combined.

LOVE THE SKIN YOU'RE IN

Skin, Hydration, Glow

This hydrating breakfast smoothie is light yet loaded with good-for-your-skin super powders, electrolytes, and healthy fats.

Makes 1 serving

½ cup coconut water
¼ cup filtered water
1 teaspoon coconut butter
½ cup raspberries or strawberries or both (frozen works great here!)
1 tablespoon collagen peptides
1 teaspoon sea buckthorn powder
¼ teaspoon Schisandra berry powder

Place all the ingredients in a blender and blend on high speed for about 1 minute, or until well combined.

RASPBERRY CHIA JAM

Antioxidant Power, Beauty, Skin Health

This delicious jam can be stirred into oats, yogurt, or spread on your favorite sourdough toast or seedy cracker. It's jam-packed (pun intended) with vitamins and skin-supporting super powders.

Makes approximately 10 ounces of jam

2 1/2 cups frozen raspberries
2 1/2 tablespoons pure maple syrup or coconut nectar
Zest and juice of 1/2 lemon
2 tablespoons chia seeds
1 teaspoon baobab powder
1 teaspoon pearl powder
1 tablespoon sea buckthorn powder

1. Place the frozen raspberries, maple syrup, and lemon zest and juice in a pot and heat over medium heat.

2. Let simmer for 7 minutes, or until the sauce is starting to thicken.

3. Remove the pot from the heat and add the chia seeds, making sure to stir well until all is well combined.

4. Place the pot back on the heat and cook for another 3 minutes.

5. Remove from the heat and let cool, then stir in the adaptogen powders.

6. Store in an airtight jar for up to 1 week.

BROTHS, SAUCES, AND BLENDS

This section is a mix of other super powder–boosted foods! Here you'll find some more savory options and easy blender sauces to keep handy and use for salads or crudités, or to upgrade any boring piece of protein or bowl of grains. There are also a few bigger-batch options for good stuff to keep on hand at all times.

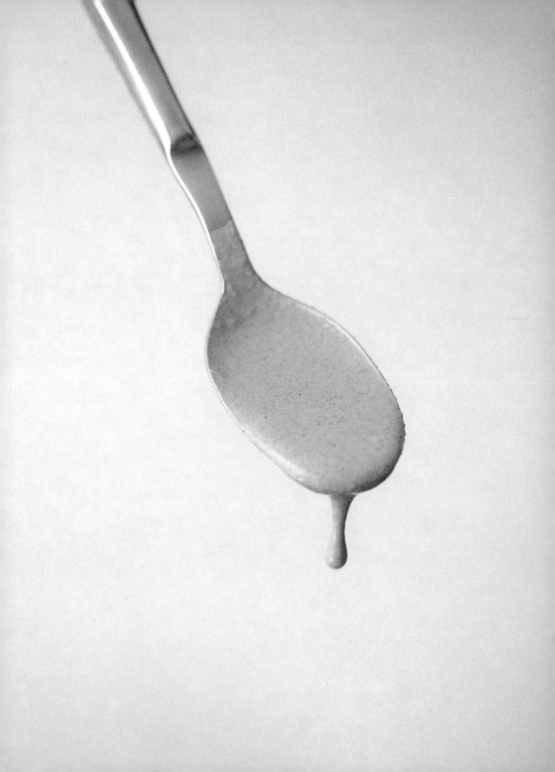

GREEN GODDESS DRESSING OR DIP

Detox, Energy, Immunity Support

Don't you worry—your vegetables will be thrilled to meet this dressing and dip. Toss your romaine or other hearty lettuces with this dressing for a delicious salad experience or pour it into a bowl alongside a tray of fresh crudités. You won't want to stop dipping. While most green goddess dressings are packed with man-made vegetable oils and dairy; this is a cleaned-up version with added green benefits!

Makes 10 ounces

½ cup avocado oil
1 tablespoon cider vinegar
1 tablespoon fresh lemon juice
2 anchovy fillets
1 garlic clove
1½ cups fresh parsley
¼ cup chopped chives
½ cup mayonnaise (I like to use Primal Kitchen or Sir Kensington—or make your own!)
¼ teaspoon freshly ground black pepper
1 teaspoon moringa leaf powder
½ teaspoon chlorella
½ teaspoon ashitaba
Sea salt, if needed

1. Place the oil, vinegar, lemon juice, anchovies, garlic, parsley, and chives in a blender.

2. Blend until smooth, 1 to 2 minutes.

3. Add the mayo, pepper, and powders and blend again until smooth.

4. Taste for saltiness (the anchovies will add salt) and season with extra sea salt as needed.

5. Serve right away for the ultimate fresh taste or store in an airtight jar in the fridge for up to 2 days.

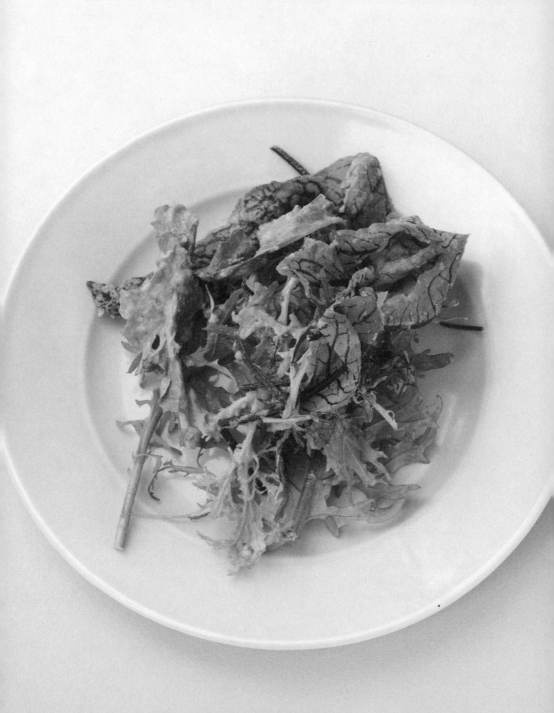

CARROT GINGER DRESSING WITH MAGIC MUSHROOMS

Digestion, Antioxidants, Immunity Support

A bright dressing you can pour over your favorite leafy greens, on top of fish, or simply use for dipping crudités! It's reminiscent of the dressing you get on your salad at your local sushi joint and is made with whole, clean foods and oils. Make a batch to keep in the fridge and you'll always have something great to elevate any platter of veggies to new heights.

Makes about 16 ounces

1½ cups chopped carrot (2-inch chunks)
2 large or 3 small shallots, quartered
¼ cup minced fresh ginger
¼ cup apple cider vinegar
2 tablespoons raw honey
3 tablespoons toasted sesame oil
2 teaspoons extra-virgin olive oil
2 tablespoons water
½ teaspoon sea salt
¼ teaspoon freshly ground black pepper
3 teaspoons reishi
3 teaspoons cordyceps
1 teaspoon lion's mane

1. Place all the ingredients in a high-speed blender or food processor.

2. Start with a lower speed and slowly increase the speed, to enable all the ingredients to blend well. Continue on high speed for 1 minute, or until smooth.

3. Pour into a jar and store in the fridge for up to a week.

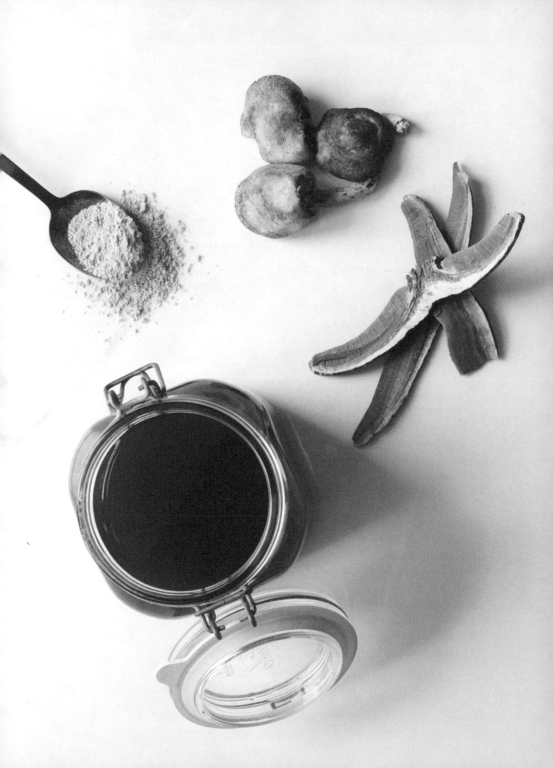

MUSHROOM BROTH

Grounding, Anti-Inflammatory, Focus

This is a comforting, grounding, and nurturing vegan broth.
Make a batch and warm up a cup at a time as a snack, a morning
brew, or a nightcap.

Makes about 1½ quarts

BROTH
1 ounce dried mushrooms
   (porcini, shiitake, maitake, or
   oyster)
2 quarts filtered or spring water
2 strips kelp
2 onions, chopped coarsely
3 carrots, chopped coarsely
2 celery stalks, chopped coarsely
1 tablespoon black peppercorns
2 bay leaves
6 sprigs thyme

**ADD (ANY OR ALL) WHEN
PREPARING A SERVING:**
1 garlic clove, finely chopped
1 teaspoon organic miso (I like
   chickpea miso)
½ teaspoon ground turmeric
1 teaspoon dulse flakes
¼ teaspoon reishi
¼ teaspoon cordyceps
¼ teaspoon chaga
¼ teaspoon lion's mane

1. Place the dried mushrooms in a bowl and cover with room-temperature water. Let sit for 20 minutes, until soft.

2. Place the filtered water in a large pot and add the kelp, onions, carrots, and celery.

3. Lift the mushrooms out of the soaking liquid and add to the broth pot.

4. Strain the soaking liquid through a fine-mesh sieve into the broth pot. Add the peppercorns, bay leaves, and thyme.

5. Bring the pot to a boil and let simmer for 90 minutes over medium heat.

6. Remove from the heat and let the broth cool, then strain through a fine-mesh sieve into a large bowl. Press on

continued

BROTHS, SAUCES, AND BLENDS

the solids to extract as much liquid as possible. Discard the solids.

7. Store in an airtight container in the fridge, or freeze in individual 1-cup portions or ice cube trays.

8. To serve, warm up a portion in a small pot.

9. Stir the garlic, miso, turmeric, dulse, reishi, cordyceps, chaga, and/or lion's mane into the serving of broth.

PUMPED-UP BONE BROTH WITH TURMERIC, GINGER, AND GHEE

Skin Health, Healing/Recovery, Immunity Boost

Bone broth has amazing gut-healing and skin- and joint-supporting benefits. You can make your own using bones from your local butcher, or buy fresh or frozen bone broth. Use that broth as your base, and mix it up with super powders, fresh spices, and good fats. A cup a day may keep the doctor away.

Makes 1 serving

1½ cups bone broth
1 garlic clove, minced finely
⅓ teaspoon ground turmeric
⅓ teaspoon ground ginger
⅛ teaspoon freshly ground
  black pepper
¼ teaspoon reishi
¼ teaspoon astragalus
1 teaspoon ghee

1. Warm up the bone broth and garlic in a small pot.

2. Place the powders in a cup or bowl, pour in the warmed broth, and stir in the ghee.

3. Sip slowly.

ADAPTOGENIC HONEY

Mood Booster, Stress Fighter, Protection

This is an easy way to add some adaptogens to your tea every day. Simply stir the powders into raw or manuka honey and then add to your next cup of tea for an elevated experience! This honey can also be drizzled on oatmeal, yogurt, or a fruit salad, or onto almond butter on toast. Use only about 1 teaspoon of the adaptogenic honey at a time to ensure you don't take too much at once.

Makes 20 servings

1 cup raw or manuka honey
5 teaspoons *Mucuna pruriens*
5 teaspoons rhodiola
2 teaspoons ashwagandha
5 teaspoons astragalus

1. Place the honey in a medium bowl, add the powders, and stir to mix well.

2. Store in an airtight jar.

GOLDEN MILK POWDER BLEND

Anti-Inflammatory, Digestive Support, Calming

A golden latte is oh so nourishing, comforting, and delicious, but it does require quite a few powders and ingredients to make. An easy shortcut is to premake a powdered blend to which you can add to a cup of warmed milk with a little honey.

Makes 80 servings

1 cup ground turmeric
3 tablespoons ground ginger
1 tablespoon freshly ground
  black pepper
1 tablespoon ground cardamom
2 tablespoons ground coriander
3 tablespoons ground star anise
1 tablespoon ground cloves
1 teaspoon ground nutmeg
4 tablespoons ground cinnamon
1 teaspoon ashwagandha
2 tablespoons vanilla powder

1. Stir all the powders together in a bowl.

2. Transfer to a lidded jar and store for whenever you want some golden milk!

3. To make golden milk, add a heaping teaspoon of the mixture to 1 cup of warm milk and stir. Add 1 teaspoon of honey or pure maple syrup (or sweeten to your taste).

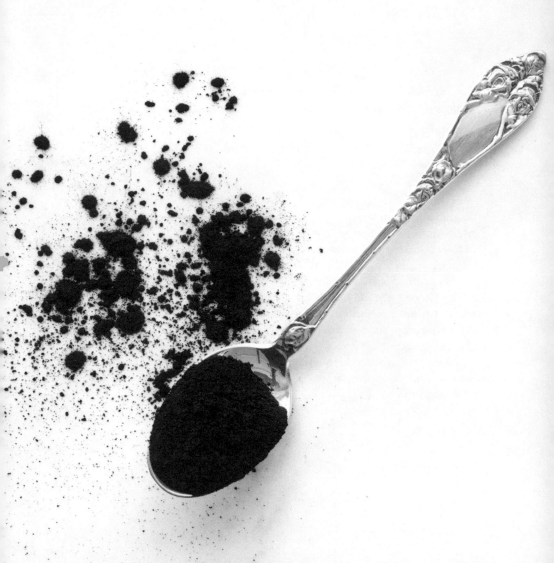

GLOSSARY

Antioxidant: a substance preventing cell damage from free radicals and oxidation. Some are found in plants, and the body itself makes some.

Adrenal glands: responsible for production and secretion of the hormones adrenaline and cortisol.

Adrenaline: a hormone secreted by the adrenal glands that increases blood circulation and breathing and prepares the muscles for exertion.

Aphrodisiac: the term used for any food or substance that stimulates sexual desire.

Ayurveda: a traditional system of wellness, or "science of life," stemming from India that incorporates herbs, body work, and diet with an emphasis on mind-body connection.

Botanical: describes a substance derived from one part of a plant. It can be the leaf, root, stem, berry, or flower.

Cortisol: often referred to as the stress hormone. It is released by the adrenal glands in response to stress.

Endocrine system: also referred to as the body's hormonal system. It's made up of glands that release their hormones directly into the bloodstream.

Herb: a plant for culinary or medicinal use that does not have a permanent stem (not a tree or a bush).

Medicinal: refers to a substance containing healing properties.

Superfood: a nutrient-dense food beneficial for health and overall well-being.

Tonic herbs: in Chinese medicine, the term *tonic* is used to describe plants that are toning and that alleviate weaknesses in the body. They are believed to increase well-being and support balance. You may see the term *liver tonic* or *qi tonic* (strengthens the immunity defenses) in literature about herbs.

ACKNOWLEDGMENTS

There are many people to thank who have made this book a reality. Thanks to Dr. Frank Lipman for introducing me to and teaching me about these amazing plants. And for his continued support and curiosity, and for being the embodiment of a growth mindset.

Thanks to David Schulze for all the amazing images in this book, for the fun times shooting them, and for his input and art direction. Thanks, too, to Steve for being there with helping hands, pots and pans, and to Talia Sparrow for introducing us and making up my face.

A big thank you to my husband, Roald, for always believing in me and believing that I'm capable of a lot more than I could ever imagine. And to my children, Felix and Freya, who are the joy of my life and inspire me to do better every day. Their endless energy and love for life is the reason this tired mamma needed to turn to these super powders in the first place. And thanks to Ana—without her I would not have found the time to research and write this book.

Thanks to Ann Treistman and Aurora Bell and their team at Countryman Press for holding my hand through this process, putting all the content together so beautifully, and for their ongoing trust and support.

INDEX

186

187

191

ABOUT THE
AUTHOR

Katrine van Wyk, the author of *Best Green Drinks Ever* and *Best Green Eats Ever*, is a certified Holistic Health Coach, and yoga teacher. She moved to New York City from Norway in 2006 to work as a model. The years of being in front of the camera, traveling, and working long hours taught her a lot about what it takes to take care of oneself and maintain a healthy lifestyle. After growing tired of the modeling industry, she left to complete her undergraduate studies at the New School in New York. Katrine then furthered her studies at the Institute for Integrative Nutrition where she was trained in more than one hundred dietary theories and studied a variety of practical lifestyle coaching methods. Katrine has since trained with Dr. Frank Lipman and now works closely with him at his practice in Manhattan, The Eleven Eleven Wellness Center. As part of Dr. Lipman's team of health coaches, Katrine has helped guide his high-profile patients through dietary changes that fit their demanding and busy lives. Katrine lives in Brooklyn with her husband and two children.